Computed Tomography Exam

SECRETS

Study Guide
Your Key to Exam Success

CT Test Review for the
Computed Tomography Exam

Dear Future Exam Success Story:

First of all, **THANK YOU** for purchasing Mometrix study materials!

Second, congratulations! You are one of the few determined test-takers who are committed to doing whatever it takes to excel on your exam. **You have come to the right place.** We developed these study materials with one goal in mind: to deliver you the information you need in a format that's concise and easy to use.

In addition to optimizing your guide for the content of the test, we've outlined our recommended steps for breaking down the preparation process into small, attainable goals so you can make sure you stay on track.

We've also analyzed the entire test-taking process, identifying the most common pitfalls and showing how you can overcome them and be ready for any curveball the test throws you.

Standardized testing is one of the biggest obstacles on your road to success, which only increases the importance of doing well in the high-pressure, high-stakes environment of test day. Your results on this test could have a significant impact on your future, and this guide provides the information and practical advice to help you achieve your full potential on test day.

Your success is our success

We would love to hear from you! If you would like to share the story of your exam success or if you have any questions or comments in regard to our products, please contact us at **800-673-8175** or **support@mometrix.com**.

Thanks again for your business and we wish you continued success!

Sincerely,
The Mometrix Test Preparation Team

Need more help? Check out our flashcards at: http://MometrixFlashcards.com/CT

Copyright © 2018 by Mometrix Media LLC. All rights reserved.
Written and edited by the Mometrix Exam Secrets Test Prep Team
Printed in the United States of America

TABLE OF CONTENTS

INTRODUCTION 1

SECRET KEY #1 – PLAN BIG, STUDY SMALL 2
    INFORMATION ORGANIZATION 2
    TIME MANAGEMENT 2
    STUDY ENVIRONMENT 2

SECRET KEY #2 – MAKE YOUR STUDYING COUNT 3
    RETENTION 3
    MODALITY 3

SECRET KEY #3 – PRACTICE THE RIGHT WAY 4
    PRACTICE TEST STRATEGY 5

SECRET KEY #4 – PACE YOURSELF 6

SECRET KEY #5 – HAVE A PLAN FOR GUESSING 7
    WHEN TO START THE GUESSING PROCESS 7
    HOW TO NARROW DOWN THE CHOICES 8
    WHICH ANSWER TO CHOOSE 9

TEST-TAKING STRATEGIES 10
    QUESTION STRATEGIES 10
    ANSWER CHOICE STRATEGIES 11
    GENERAL STRATEGIES 12
    FINAL NOTES 13

PATIENT CARE 15
    PATIENT PREPARATION 15
    ASSESSMENT AND MONITORING 16
    IV PROCEDURES 17
    CONTRAST AGENTS 19
    RADIATION SAFETY AND DOSIMETRY 24

IMAGING PROCEDURES 29
    TYPE OF STUDY 29
    FOCUS OF QUESTIONS 47

PHYSICS AND INSTRUMENTATION 63
    SYSTEM PRINCIPLES, OPERATION AND COMPONENTS 63
    IMAGE PROCESSING AND DISPLAY 67
    IMAGE QUALITY 75
    ARTIFACT RECOGNITION AND REDUCTION 79

IMPORTANT TERMS 82

CT PRACTICE TEST 91

ANSWER KEY AND EXPLANATIONS 119

HOW TO OVERCOME TEST ANXIETY 138
    CAUSES OF TEST ANXIETY 138
    ELEMENTS OF TEST ANXIETY 139
    EFFECTS OF TEST ANXIETY 139
    PHYSICAL STEPS FOR BEATING TEST ANXIETY 140

    Mental Steps for Beating Test Anxiety 141
    Study Strategy 142
    Test Tips 144
    Important Qualification 145

THANK YOU **146**

ADDITIONAL BONUS MATERIAL **147**

Introduction

Thank you for purchasing this resource! You have made the choice to prepare yourself for a test that could have a huge impact on your future, and this guide is designed to help you be fully ready for test day. Obviously, it's important to have a solid understanding of the test material, but you also need to be prepared for the unique environment and stressors of the test, so that you can perform to the best of your abilities.

For this purpose, the first section that appears in this guide is the **Secret Keys**. We've devoted countless hours to meticulously researching what works and what doesn't, and we've boiled down our findings to the five most impactful steps you can take to improve your performance on the test. We start at the beginning with study planning and move through the preparation process, all the way to the testing strategies that will help you get the most out of what you know when you're finally sitting in front of the test.

We recommend that you start preparing for your test as far in advance as possible. However, if you've bought this guide as a last-minute study resource and only have a few days before your test, we recommend that you skip over the first two Secret Keys since they address a long-term study plan.

If you struggle with **test anxiety**, we strongly encourage you to check out our recommendations for how you can overcome it. Test anxiety is a formidable foe, but it can be beaten, and we want to make sure you have the tools you need to defeat it.

Secret Key #1 – Plan Big, Study Small

There's a lot riding on your performance. If you want to ace this test, you're going to need to keep your skills sharp and the material fresh in your mind. You need a plan that lets you review everything you need to know while still fitting in your schedule. We'll break this strategy down into three categories.

Information Organization

Start with the information you already have: the official test outline. From this, you can make a complete list of all the concepts you need to cover before the test. Organize these concepts into groups that can be studied together, and create a list of any related vocabulary you need to learn so you can brush up on any difficult terms. You'll want to keep this vocabulary list handy once you actually start studying since you may need to add to it along the way.

Time Management

Once you have your set of study concepts, decide how to spread them out over the time you have left before the test. Break your study plan into small, clear goals so you have a manageable task for each day and know exactly what you're doing. Then just focus on one small step at a time. When you manage your time this way, you don't need to spend hours at a time studying. Studying a small block of content for a short period each day helps you retain information better and avoid stressing over how much you have left to do. You can relax knowing that you have a plan to cover everything in time. In order for this strategy to be effective though, you have to start studying early and stick to your schedule. Avoid the exhaustion and futility that comes from last-minute cramming!

Study Environment

The environment you study in has a big impact on your learning. Studying in a coffee shop, while probably more enjoyable, is not likely to be as fruitful as studying in a quiet room. It's important to keep distractions to a minimum. You're only planning to study for a short block of time, so make the most of it. Don't pause to check your phone or get up to find a snack. It's also important to **avoid multitasking**. Research has consistently shown that multitasking will make your studying dramatically less effective. Your study area should also be comfortable and well-lit so you don't have the distraction of straining your eyes or sitting on an uncomfortable chair.

The time of day you study is also important. You want to be rested and alert. Don't wait until just before bedtime. Study when you'll be most likely to comprehend and remember. Even better, if you know what time of day your test will be, set that time aside for study. That way your brain will be used to working on that subject at that specific time and you'll have a better chance of recalling information.

Finally, it can be helpful to team up with others who are studying for the same test. Your actual studying should be done in as isolated an environment as possible, but the work of organizing the information and setting up the study plan can be divided up. In between study sessions, you can discuss with your teammates the concepts that you're all studying and quiz each other on the details. Just be sure that your teammates are as serious about the test as you are. If you find that your study time is being replaced with social time, you might need to find a new team.

Secret Key #2 – Make Your Studying Count

You're devoting a lot of time and effort to preparing for this test, so you want to be absolutely certain it will pay off. This means doing more than just reading the content and hoping you can remember it on test day. It's important to make every minute of study count. There are two main areas you can focus on to make your studying count:

Retention

It doesn't matter how much time you study if you can't remember the material. You need to make sure you are retaining the concepts. To check your retention of the information you're learning, try recalling it at later times with minimal prompting. Try carrying around flashcards and glance at one or two from time to time or ask a friend who's also studying for the test to quiz you.

To enhance your retention, look for ways to put the information into practice so that you can apply it rather than simply recalling it. If you're using the information in practical ways, it will be much easier to remember. Similarly, it helps to solidify a concept in your mind if you're not only reading it to yourself but also explaining it to someone else. Ask a friend to let you teach them about a concept you're a little shaky on (or speak aloud to an imaginary audience if necessary). As you try to summarize, define, give examples, and answer your friend's questions, you'll understand the concepts better and they will stay with you longer. Finally, step back for a big picture view and ask yourself how each piece of information fits with the whole subject. When you link the different concepts together and see them working together as a whole, it's easier to remember the individual components.

Finally, practice showing your work on any multi-step problems, even if you're just studying. Writing out each step you take to solve a problem will help solidify the process in your mind, and you'll be more likely to remember it during the test.

Modality

Modality simply refers to the means or method by which you study. Choosing a study modality that fits your own individual learning style is crucial. No two people learn best in exactly the same way, so it's important to know your strengths and use them to your advantage.

For example, if you learn best by visualization, focus on visualizing a concept in your mind and draw an image or a diagram. Try color-coding your notes, illustrating them, or creating symbols that will trigger your mind to recall a learned concept. If you learn best by hearing or discussing information, find a study partner who learns the same way or read aloud to yourself. Think about how to put the information in your own words. Imagine that you are giving a lecture on the topic and record yourself so you can listen to it later.

For any learning style, flashcards can be helpful. Organize the information so you can take advantage of spare moments to review. Underline key words or phrases. Use different colors for different categories. Mnemonic devices (such as creating a short list in which every item starts with the same letter) can also help with retention. Find what works best for you and use it to store the information in your mind most effectively and easily.

Secret Key #3 – Practice the Right Way

Your success on test day depends not only on how many hours you put into preparing, but also on whether you prepared the right way. It's good to check along the way to see if your studying is paying off. One of the most effective ways to do this is by taking practice tests to evaluate your progress. Practice tests are useful because they show exactly where you need to improve. Every time you take a practice test, pay special attention to these three groups of questions:

- The questions you got wrong
- The questions you had to guess on, even if you guessed right
- The questions you found difficult or slow to work through

This will show you exactly what your weak areas are, and where you need to devote more study time. Ask yourself why each of these questions gave you trouble. Was it because you didn't understand the material? Was it because you didn't remember the vocabulary? Do you need more repetitions on this type of question to build speed and confidence? Dig into those questions and figure out how you can strengthen your weak areas as you go back to review the material.

Additionally, many practice tests have a section explaining the answer choices. It can be tempting to read the explanation and think that you now have a good understanding of the concept. However, an explanation likely only covers part of the question's broader context. Even if the explanation makes sense, **go back and investigate** every concept related to the question until you're positive you have a thorough understanding.

As you go along, keep in mind that the practice test is just that: practice. Memorizing these questions and answers will not be very helpful on the actual test because it is unlikely to have any of the same exact questions. If you only know the right answers to the sample questions, you won't be prepared for the real thing. **Study the concepts** until you understand them fully, and then you'll be able to answer any question that shows up on the test.

It's important to wait on the practice tests until you're ready. If you take a test on your first day of study, you may be overwhelmed by the amount of material covered and how much you need to learn. Work up to it gradually.

On test day, you'll need to be prepared for answering questions, managing your time, and using the test-taking strategies you've learned. It's a lot to balance, like a mental marathon that will have a big impact on your future. Like training for a marathon, you'll need to start slowly and work your way up. When test day arrives, you'll be ready.

Start with the strategies you've read in the first two Secret Keys—plan your course and study in the way that works best for you. If you have time, consider using multiple study resources to get different approaches to the same concepts. It can be helpful to see difficult concepts from more than one angle. Then find a good source for practice tests. Many times, the test website will suggest potential study resources or provide sample tests.

Practice Test Strategy

When you're ready to start taking practice tests, follow this strategy:

1. Take the first test with no time constraints and with your notes and study guide handy. Take your time and focus on applying the strategies you've learned.
2. Take the second practice test open-book as well, but set a timer and practice pacing yourself to finish in time.
3. Take any other practice tests as if it were test day. Set a timer and put away your study materials. Sit at a table or desk in a quiet room, imagine yourself at the testing center, and answer questions as quickly and accurately as possible.
4. Keep repeating step 3 on a regular basis until you run out of practice tests or it's time for the actual test. Your mind will be ready for the schedule and stress of test day, and you'll be able to focus on recalling the material you've learned.

Secret Key #4 – Pace Yourself

Once you're fully prepared for the material on the test, your biggest challenge on test day will be managing your time. Just knowing that the clock is ticking can make you panic even if you have plenty of time left. Work on pacing yourself so you can build confidence against the time constraints of the exam. Pacing is a difficult skill to master, especially in a high-pressure environment, so **practice is vital**.

Set time expectations for your pace based on how much time is available. For example, if a section has 60 questions and the time limit is 30 minutes, you know you have to average 30 seconds or less per question in order to answer them all. Although 30 seconds is the hard limit, set 25 seconds per question as your goal, so you reserve extra time to spend on harder questions. When you budget extra time for the harder questions, you no longer have any reason to stress when those questions take longer to answer.

Don't let this time expectation distract you from working through the test at a calm, steady pace, but keep it in mind so you don't spend too much time on any one question. Recognize that taking extra time on one question you don't understand may keep you from answering two that you do understand later in the test. If your time limit for a question is up and you're still not sure of the answer, mark it and move on, and come back to it later if the time and the test format allow. If the testing format doesn't allow you to return to earlier questions, just make an educated guess; then put it out of your mind and move on.

On the easier questions, be careful not to rush. It may seem wise to hurry through them so you have more time for the challenging ones, but it's not worth missing one if you know the concept and just didn't take the time to read the question fully. Work efficiently but make sure you understand the question and have looked at all of the answer choices, since more than one may seem right at first.

Even if you're paying attention to the time, you may find yourself a little behind at some point. You should speed up to get back on track, but do so wisely. Don't panic; just take a few seconds less on each question until you're caught up. Don't guess without thinking, but do look through the answer choices and eliminate any you know are wrong. If you can get down to two choices, it is often worthwhile to guess from those. Once you've chosen an answer, move on and don't dwell on any that you skipped or had to hurry through. If a question was taking too long, chances are it was one of the harder ones, so you weren't as likely to get it right anyway.

On the other hand, if you find yourself getting ahead of schedule, it may be beneficial to slow down a little. The more quickly you work, the more likely you are to make a careless mistake that will affect your score. You've budgeted time for each question, so don't be afraid to spend that time. Practice an efficient but careful pace to get the most out of the time you have.

Secret Key #5 – Have a Plan for Guessing

When you're taking the test, you may find yourself stuck on a question. Some of the answer choices seem better than others, but you don't see the one answer choice that is obviously correct. What do you do?

The scenario described above is very common, yet most test takers have not effectively prepared for it. Developing and practicing a plan for guessing may be one of the single most effective uses of your time as you get ready for the exam.

In developing your plan for guessing, there are three questions to address:

- When should you start the guessing process?
- How should you narrow down the choices?
- Which answer should you choose?

When to Start the Guessing Process

Unless your plan for guessing is to select C every time (which, despite its merits, is not what we recommend), you need to leave yourself enough time to apply your answer elimination strategies. Since you have a limited amount of time for each question, that means that if you're going to give yourself the best shot at guessing correctly, you have to decide quickly whether or not you will guess.

Of course, the best-case scenario is that you don't have to guess at all, so first, see if you can answer the question based on your knowledge of the subject and basic reasoning skills. Focus on the key words in the question and try to jog your memory of related topics. Give yourself a chance to bring the knowledge to mind, but once you realize that you don't have (or you can't access) the knowledge you need to answer the question, it's time to start the guessing process.

It's almost always better to start the guessing process too early than too late. It only takes a few seconds to remember something and answer the question from knowledge. Carefully eliminating wrong answer choices takes longer. Plus, going through the process of eliminating answer choices can actually help jog your memory.

Summary: Start the guessing process as soon as you decide that you can't answer the question based on your knowledge.

How to Narrow Down the Choices

The next chapter in this book (**Test-Taking Strategies**) includes a wide range of strategies for how to approach questions and how to look for answer choices to eliminate. You will definitely want to read those carefully, practice them, and figure out which ones work best for you. Here though, we're going to address a mindset rather than a particular strategy.

Your chances of guessing an answer correctly depend on how many options you are choosing from.

How many choices you have	How likely you are to guess correctly
5	20%
4	25%
3	33%
2	50%
1	100%

You can see from this chart just how valuable it is to be able to eliminate incorrect answers and make an educated guess, but there are two things that many test takers do that cause them to miss out on the benefits of guessing:

- Accidentally eliminating the correct answer
- Selecting an answer based on an impression

We'll look at the first one here, and the second one in the next section.

To avoid accidentally eliminating the correct answer, we recommend a thought exercise called **the $5 challenge**. In this challenge, you only eliminate an answer choice from contention if you are willing to bet $5 on it being wrong. Why $5? Five dollars is a small but not insignificant amount of money. It's an amount you could afford to lose but wouldn't want to throw away. And while losing $5 once might not hurt too much, doing it twenty times will set you back $100. In the same way, each small decision you make—eliminating a choice here, guessing on a question there—won't by itself impact your score very much, but when you put them all together, they can make a big difference. By holding each answer choice elimination decision to a higher standard, you can reduce the risk of accidentally eliminating the correct answer.

The $5 challenge can also be applied in a positive sense: If you are willing to bet $5 that an answer choice *is* correct, go ahead and mark it as correct.

Summary: Only eliminate an answer choice if you are willing to bet $5 that it is wrong.

Which Answer to Choose

You're taking the test. You've run into a hard question and decided you'll have to guess. You've eliminated all the answer choices you're willing to bet $5 on. Now you have to pick an answer. Why do we even need to talk about this? Why can't you just pick whichever one you feel like when the time comes?

The answer to these questions is that if you don't come into the test with a plan, you'll rely on your impression to select an answer choice, and if you do that, you risk falling into a trap. The test writers know that everyone who takes their test will be guessing on some of the questions, so they intentionally write wrong answer choices to seem plausible. You still have to pick an answer though, and if the wrong answer choices are designed to look right, how can you ever be sure that you're not falling for their trap? The best solution we've found to this dilemma is to take the decision out of your hands entirely. Here is the process we recommend:

Once you've eliminated any choices that you are confident (willing to bet $5) are wrong, select the first remaining choice as your answer.

Whether you choose to select the first remaining choice, the second, or the last, the important thing is that you use some preselected standard. Using this approach guarantees that you will not be enticed into selecting an answer choice that looks right, because you are not basing your decision on how the answer choices look.

This is not meant to make you question your knowledge. Instead, it is to help you recognize the difference between your knowledge and your impressions. There's a huge difference between thinking an answer is right because of what you know, and thinking an answer is right because it looks or sounds like it should be right.

Summary: To ensure that your selection is appropriately random, make a predetermined selection from among all answer choices you have not eliminated.

Test-Taking Strategies

This section contains a list of test-taking strategies that you may find helpful as you work through the test. By taking what you know and applying logical thought, you can maximize your chances of answering any question correctly!

It is very important to realize that every question is different and every person is different: no single strategy will work on every question, and no single strategy will work for every person. That's why we've included all of them here, so you can try them out and determine which ones work best for different types of questions and which ones work best for you.

Question Strategies

Read Carefully

Read the question and answer choices carefully. Don't miss the question because you misread the terms. You have plenty of time to read each question thoroughly and make sure you understand what is being asked. Yet a happy medium must be attained, so don't waste too much time. You must read carefully, but efficiently.

Contextual Clues

Look for contextual clues. If the question includes a word you are not familiar with, look at the immediate context for some indication of what the word might mean. Contextual clues can often give you all the information you need to decipher the meaning of an unfamiliar word. Even if you can't determine the meaning, you may be able to narrow down the possibilities enough to make a solid guess at the answer to the question.

Prefixes

If you're having trouble with a word in the question or answer choices, try dissecting it. Take advantage of every clue that the word might include. Prefixes and suffixes can be a huge help. Usually they allow you to determine a basic meaning. Pre- means before, post- means after, pro - is positive, de- is negative. From prefixes and suffixes, you can get an idea of the general meaning of the word and try to put it into context.

Hedge Words

Watch out for critical hedge words, such as *likely, may, can, sometimes, often, almost, mostly, usually, generally, rarely,* and *sometimes*. Question writers insert these hedge phrases to cover every possibility. Often an answer choice will be wrong simply because it leaves no room for exception. Be on guard for answer choices that have definitive words such as *exactly* and *always*.

Switchback Words

Stay alert for *switchbacks*. These are the words and phrases frequently used to alert you to shifts in thought. The most common switchback words are *but, although*, and *however*. Others include *nevertheless, on the other hand, even though, while, in spite of, despite, regardless of*. Switchback words are important to catch because they can change the direction of the question or an answer choice.

Face Value

When in doubt, use common sense. Accept the situation in the problem at face value. Don't read too much into it. These problems will not require you to make wild assumptions. If you have to go beyond creativity and warp time or space in order to have an answer choice fit the question, then you should move on and consider the other answer choices. These are normal problems rooted in reality. The applicable relationship or explanation may not be readily apparent, but it is there for you to figure out. Use your common sense to interpret anything that isn't clear.

Answer Choice Strategies

Answer Selection

The most thorough way to pick an answer choice is to identify and eliminate wrong answers until only one is left, then confirm it is the correct answer. Sometimes an answer choice may immediately seem right, but be careful. The test writers will usually put more than one reasonable answer choice on each question, so take a second to read all of them and make sure that the other choices are not equally obvious. As long as you have time left, it is better to read every answer choice than to pick the first one that looks right without checking the others.

Answer Choice Families

An answer choice family consists of two (in rare cases, three) answer choices that are very similar in construction and cannot all be true at the same time. If you see two answer choices that are direct opposites or parallels, one of them is usually the correct answer. For instance, if one answer choice says that quantity x increases and another either says that quantity x decreases (opposite) or says that quantity y increases (parallel), then those answer choices would fall into the same family. An answer choice that doesn't match the construction of the answer choice family is more likely to be incorrect. Most questions will not have answer choice families, but when they do appear, you should be prepared to recognize them.

Eliminate Answers

Eliminate answer choices as soon as you realize they are wrong, but make sure you consider all possibilities. If you are eliminating answer choices and realize that the last one you are left with is also wrong, don't panic. Start over and consider each choice again. There may be something you missed the first time that you will realize on the second pass.

Avoid Fact Traps

Don't be distracted by an answer choice that is factually true but doesn't answer the question. You are looking for the choice that answers the question. Stay focused on what the question is asking for so you don't accidentally pick an answer that is true but incorrect. Always go back to the question and make sure the answer choice you've selected actually answers the question and is not merely a true statement.

Extreme Statements

In general, you should avoid answers that put forth extreme actions as standard practice or proclaim controversial ideas as established fact. An answer choice that states the "process should be used in certain situations, if..." is much more likely to be correct than one that states the "process should be discontinued completely." The first is a calm rational statement and doesn't even make a definitive, uncompromising stance, using a hedge word *if* to provide wiggle room, whereas the second choice is a radical idea and far more extreme.

Benchmark

As you read through the answer choices and you come across one that seems to answer the question well, mentally select that answer choice. This is not your final answer, but it's the one that will help you evaluate the other answer choices. The one that you selected is your benchmark or standard for judging each of the other answer choices. Every other answer choice must be compared to your benchmark. That choice is correct until proven otherwise by another answer choice beating it. If you find a better answer, then that one becomes your new benchmark. Once you've decided that no other choice answers the question as well as your benchmark, you have your final answer.

Predict the Answer

Before you even start looking at the answer choices, it is often best to try to predict the answer. When you come up with the answer on your own, it is easier to avoid distractions and traps because you will know exactly what to look for. The right answer choice is unlikely to be word-for-word what you came up with, but it should be a close match. Even if you are confident that you have the right answer, you should still take the time to read each option before moving on.

General Strategies

Tough Questions

If you are stumped on a problem or it appears too hard or too difficult, don't waste time. Move on! Remember though, if you can quickly check for obviously incorrect answer choices, your chances of guessing correctly are greatly improved. Before you completely give up, at least try to knock out a couple of possible answers. Eliminate what you can and then guess at the remaining answer choices before moving on.

Check Your Work

Since you will probably not know every term listed and the answer to every question, it is important that you get credit for the ones that you do know. Don't miss any questions through careless mistakes. If at all possible, try to take a second to look back over your answer selection and make sure you've selected the correct answer choice and haven't made a costly careless mistake (such as marking an answer choice that you didn't mean to mark). This quick double check should more than pay for itself in caught mistakes for the time it costs.

Pace Yourself

It's easy to be overwhelmed when you're looking at a page full of questions; your mind is confused and full of random thoughts, and the clock is ticking down faster than you would like. Calm down and maintain the pace that you have set for yourself. Especially as you get down to the last few minutes of the test, don't let the small numbers on the clock make you panic. As long as you are on track by monitoring your pace, you are guaranteed to have time for each question.

Don't Rush

It is very easy to make errors when you are in a hurry. Maintaining a fast pace in answering questions is pointless if it makes you miss questions that you would have gotten right otherwise. Test writers like to include distracting information and wrong answers that seem right. Taking a little extra time to avoid careless mistakes can make all the difference in your test score. Find a pace that allows you to be confident in the answers that you select.

Keep Moving

Panicking will not help you pass the test, so do your best to stay calm and keep moving. Taking deep breaths and going through the answer elimination steps you practiced can help to break through a stress barrier and keep your pace.

Final Notes

The combination of a solid foundation of content knowledge and the confidence that comes from practicing your plan for applying that knowledge is the key to maximizing your performance on test day. As your foundation of content knowledge is built up and strengthened, you'll find that the strategies included in this chapter become more and more effective in helping you quickly sift through the distractions and traps of the test to isolate the correct answer.

Now it's time to move on to the test content chapters of this book, but be sure to keep your goal in mind. As you read, think about how you will be able to apply this information on the test. If you've already seen sample questions for the test and you have an idea of the question format and style, try to come up with questions of your own that you can answer based on what you're reading. This will give you valuable practice applying your knowledge in the same ways you can expect to on test day.

Good luck and good studying!

Patient Care

Patient Preparation

Informed consent

The administration of any examination, especially one that has the expected complexity of computed tomography (CT), should not be performed without the informed consent of the patient and family members or caregivers, if applicable. Practitioners should attach a copy of this informed consent documentation to the medical record for auditing reasons and to prevent any legal actions should the parameters of the testing negatively affect the patient. The professional standards of conduct or other comparable guidelines of most medical facilities require the completion and proper filing of informed consent documentation before any testing. Adherence to these guidelines is considered ethical and within the limits of the law.

Scheduling and screening

Most medical facilities have employees who coordinate the scheduling of the test and the availability of the practitioner who will be performing the screening. An initial low-dose test is performed to test the patient for the baseline screening 18, and the patient is informed about the radiation dose, carcinogenic effects, and other specific information related to the benefits and risks of testing. Some facilities provide this information in a brochure with the consent form that must be completed before testing. Contact information and details about any indications or contraindications are obtained by the coordinator during the scheduling interview before administration of the test. If necessary, follow-up appointments or repeated screenings can also be scheduled.

Patient education

Practitioners should educate the patient about what to expect during the CT scan (also referred to as computerized axial tomography [CAT], computerized transaxial tomography [CTAT], or digital axial tomography [DAT]). Patients should be informed that a digital image is produced by sending x-rays through the patient. The CT scan exposes the patient to slightly more radiation than typical chest radiography, but the quality of the enhanced picture outweighs this risk. CT images provide more contrast resolution than radiographic images, and emission CT uses gamma-ray emissions and nuclear medicine from a patient who has been given a radionuclide agent before the scan. The scatter radiation associated with CT scanning reduces the radiographic contrast resolution, thereby allowing for an image with no superimposition of tissues. The CT scan produces a three-dimensional image and can provide a bone mineral assay. Some CT scans may produce false-negative findings; in such cases, the practitioner may repeat the CT scan or suggest a different type of imaging test.

Immobilization

The positioning and immobilization of the patient during CT is crucial if the practitioner is to obtain an accurate reading. The positioning should be conducive to replication because the treatment machine can reproduce the virtual simulation parameters in the event that a follow-up or second screening becomes necessary. Devices provided for immobilization and registered to the treatment table allow practitioners to position the patient correctly for the different scans required for each study, usually ranging from 100 to 200 scans. Diagnostic CT scanners are fitted with external laser alignment systems and virtual simulation software that allow practitioners to study the patient from a beam's eye view (BEV) and a room's eye view (REV) display. Digitally reconstructed radiographs (DRRs), multiplanar reformatted images (MPRs), and digitally composited radiographs (DCRs) can also be produced by the CT scanner, although these technological advances are not useful if the patient is not properly immobilized during the test.

Assessment and Monitoring

History

Before the CT scan is initiated, patients should be questioned about the occurrence of certain conditions or circumstances that may prevent the completion of the test and may endanger the patient's health. For example, patients should be questioned about allergies to iodine dye or any other substance containing iodine, as well as whether they have asthma, have allergies to any medication, or have experienced allergic reactions to bee stings or shellfish. They should also be asked whether they have any heart condition, have used metformin (Glucophage) to control diabetes, have a history of kidney problems, are pregnant or claustrophobic, have used bismuth medications within the past 4 days, or have undergone x-ray tests using barium contrast dyes. Patients may be required to ingest a contrast dye; if so, they may need to have an enema or take a laxative before testing.

<u>Kidney problems</u>

Patients with a history of kidney problems may be susceptible to irritation and damage as a result of the contrast dye used during CT scanning. Certain blood tests, specifically analyses of creatinine and blood urea nitrogen concentrations, can be completed before CT scanning so that the functionality of the kidneys can be verified and any necessary modifications to the test can be made in advance.

<u>Claustrophobia</u>

Patients who are claustrophobic or who become nervous in confined spaces may require medication for relaxation so that they can lie still inside the CT scanner. Because patients' faces are not covered, they can view the room without moving their heads and compromising the testing.

Vital signs

The machinery used to perform CT often includes provisions for monitoring the patient's vital signs, such as blood pressure, heart rate, oral temperature, and oxygen saturation. The test can be more effective if these vital signs are kept within normal limits, and doctors can choose to discontinue testing if the vital signs vary from those normal limits in response to the contrast agent, the duration of the test, or other factors. Patients are usually requested not to eat or drink for at least 4 hours before testing, although this requirement may be waived in an emergency. Patients should also be informed about immobilization on a hard table, venipuncture, a salty taste in the mouth, redness of skin during dye injection, mild nausea, diarrhea, and allergic reaction or kidney failure, which occur only rarely. Some patients are given a sedative for relaxation and easing of claustrophobia.

> **Review Video: Vital Signs**
> Visit mometrix.com/academy and enter code: 330799

Laboratory tests

In addition to the possible allergic reactions that patients may experience in response to the contrast agents used during CT scanning, other abnormal laboratory values should be considered.

- Blood urea nitrogen (BUN) is a waste product that forms in the liver and collects throughout the body in the bloodstream; the BUN concentration may be high in patients with kidney failure.
- The concentration of creatinine, a waste product found in the serum and produced by the kidneys, can be measured by a creatinine clearance test that compares the creatinine concentration in a blood sample against a formula based on the patient's sex, weight, and age.
- Prothrombin time (PT) tests measure the clotting time associated with prothrombin, the plasma protein that precedes thrombin and is involved in coagulation. PT is also an indicator of other bleeding disorders and liver damage and is used to monitor the use of anticoagulant medicines.
- Partial thromboplastin time (PTT) and platelet count should also be measured, because they relate to coagulation.

Medications

Diabetes

Patients with diabetes should be asked whether they take metformin (Glucophage). The doctor may request that the patient discontinue the use of metformin a few days before testing and then begin retaking the prescribed medication a few days after completion of the test.

IV Procedures

Venipuncture

Several important factors must be considered during the performance of venipuncture, or surgical puncture of a vein, for drawing blood or administering intravenous medication. The common veins used for such administration should be located before venipuncture is performed, and all necessary equipment and departmental pharmaceuticals should be readily available. These pharmaceuticals may include iodine-based contrast material, such as ionic and nonionic contrast dyes; high osmolar and low osmolar contrast agents, which are associated with adverse effects, precautions, dose requirements, varying susceptibility of body parts to the contrast, and peak opacification time; and sedation agents, which are associated with adverse effects, precautions, and dose requirements. The appropriate site must be selected and prepared for venipuncture, and the practitioner must insert and remove the needle correctly.

Aseptic and sterile techniques

During the physical act of administering medication, the practitioner should be aware of the basic tenets of sterilization. The medication or contrast agent must be injected with consideration for power injectors, other comparable methods, extravasation and treatment, and use of an IV pump. Any adverse reactions to contrast dyes, latex, or sedation and the treatment required for such reactions should be analyzed and included in the patient's documentation. The practitioner should always adhere to aseptic techniques and should verify that the area is free of pathogenic microorganisms so that infection can be prevented, according to the standards and guidelines set forth by the medical facility in which the venipuncture is being performed. All medical facilities must meet certain health codes regarding asepsis.

Sterile technique, method 1: The practitioner should scrub a selected area for 30 seconds with a sterile swab that is saturated in a 0.7% aqueous scrub solution of iodophor compound; any excess foam should be removed with another sterile swab. The iodophor complex solution should be applied with a sterile swab beginning at the intended venipuncture site and using gradually increasing concentric circles until an area 3 inches in diameter has been covered. The solution should be allowed to stand for 30 seconds before venipuncture is completed. If the practitioner cannot complete the venipuncture immediately after the 30-second waiting period, then the area should be covered with dry sterile gauze. If the arm is bent or the prepared site is touched by fingers or any other nonsterile object, the entire procedure for sterilization must be repeated.

Sterile technique, method 2: Another method of administering contrast agents requires scrubbing a selected area for 30 seconds with a sterile swab that is saturated in nonalcoholic, 15% aqueous soap or detergent solution so that any fat, oils, extra skin cells, dirt, and other debris can be cleaned away. The soap froth can be removed with another sterile swab saturated in 10% acetone in 70% isopropyl alcohol. The site should then be allowed to dry. A tincture of iodine can be applied with another sterile swab beginning at the venipuncture site and using gradually increasing concentric circles until an area 3 inches in diameter has been covered. The site should then be allowed to dry. The iodine can be removed with a sterile swab saturated in 10% acetone in 70% isopropyl alcohol, which should be allowed to dry. The prepared area should be covered with dry sterile gauze if the venipuncture is not completed immediately. If the arm is bent or the site is contaminated, the entire procedure must be repeated.

Sterile technique, method 3: For patients sensitive to iodine, the practitioner can directly apply 1 mL (an amount approximately the size of a penny) of One Step Gel to the venipuncture site. Held at an angle of approximately 30°, the sterile applicator can be used to scrub in a circular motion for 30 seconds until an area 1 inch in diameter directly over the venipuncture site has been covered. The same applicator can then be used, beginning at the intended venipuncture site and using gradually increasing concentric circles, to cover an area 3 inches in diameter. A second sterile applicator can be used to remove excess gel, beginning at the center of the 3-inch area and using gradually increasing concentric circles. The site should be allowed to dry according to the manufacturer's instructions. If the practitioner cannot complete the venipuncture immediately, the area should be covered with dry sterile gauze. If the arm is bent or the site is otherwise contaminated, the entire procedure must be repeated.

Sterile technique, method 4: Method 4 is the only method for sterilization of the intended injection site that does not require application in gradually increasing concentric circles from the intended venipuncture site. A solution of 2% chlorhexidine gluconate in 70% isopropyl alcohol should be prepared in advance. The practitioner should scrub the intended site of venipuncture with this solution, making repeated back-and-forth strokes across an area 2.5 inches by 2.5 inches for a minimum of 30 seconds. This repeated motion should ensure that the area is completely wet with the antiseptic. The area should be allowed to air dry for at least 30 seconds. If the practitioner cannot complete the venipuncture immediately, then the area should be covered with dry sterile gauze. If the arm is bent or the site is otherwise contaminated, the entire procedure must be repeated.

Sterile solutions in bulk: Single-use, prepackaged products can be replaced with bulk solutions in certain situations. Practitioners cannot sterilize the antiseptic solutions used to prepare the patient's arm, but these solutions can be purchased and prepared in bulk and will last for several months with proper handling. Certain solutions contain additives such as alcohol or iodophor compound that can prevent the growth of organisms. Bulk products requiring dilution should be handled in small batches at a time. Bottles of iodine solutions purchased in bulk should be tightly sealed or capped when not being used in venipuncture preparation, because alcohol evaporates over time. This potential evaporation could increase the concentration of iodine, thereby resulting in skin irritation.

Injection techniques

Either power injection or manual injection can be used to administer intravenous contrast material, although power injection provides uniformity of enhancement and allows the practitioner to verify the precise timing of the delivery of contrast materials.

- Power injection is most often used with intravenous catheters so that the injection site can be closely monitored during the initial injection and the risk of extravasation can be minimized. The flow rate should be set so that the entire amount of contrast material can be delivered over a period determined to be equal to or slightly less than that required for CT acquisition.
- Manual injection is preferred when intravenous access is achieved through a catheter located in the dorsum of the hand or wrist. If the catheter is properly positioned and well-functioning, the complications associated with both methods of injection are similar.

Pediatric patients

Power and manual injections can be used almost interchangeably for most patients, although the appropriateness of power injection involving a 24-gauge peripheral catheter has not been well established for infants and children. With proper intravascular positioning of the access, power injection can be safe for pediatric patients as long as the return of blood and the delivery of saline flush or cleansing are unimpeded. With contrast material delivered at 1.0 mL/sec, many medical facilities are seeing improvements in power injections for pediatric populations when the injection occurs through central venous access if peripheral access is unavailable.

Automatic injection

Automatic injection methods include the bolus method, in which the solution is automatically provided over a short period of time; the gravity infusion method, in which the bag of solution is connected to the tubing and needle and is administered with a timer; and the infusion pump method, in which an electronic control determines the rate and volume of the solution being injected. Automatic injection techniques are programmed for single-phase injection or multi-phase injection as determined by the power of the energy being released. The flow rate for those injections is determined by the density of the solution, the amount of time needed to administer the entire solution, and the comparable amount of time required to complete the CT scan.

Contrast Agents

Contrast agents

The efficacy of the CT scan is determined by the kind of contrast agent used to allow practitioners to more accurately view the particular body part to be analyzed. The contrast agent consists of a dye that usually contains iodine and is injected intravenously during CT scanning. This dye renders the blood vessels and other structures and organs more visible on the CT image, and the contrast agent can help practitioners evaluate blood flow, detect tumors, and locate specific areas of inflammation. Intravenous contrast agents are usually used for chest, pelvic, and abdominal CT scanning; for spinal scans, the contrast dye can be injected into the area around the spinal cord. CT images are often obtained both before and after the injection of contrast material.

Types of contrast materials

Materials are used during radiography, ultrasonography, nuclear imaging, and magnetic resonance imaging so that practitioners can view the target organ and surrounding tissue without performing open surgery and can thereby analyze the current condition of the patient's internal organs. Current research on contrast materials focuses either on developing new types of agents, thereby allowing easier and safer diagnosis, or on modifying current agents to reduce their impact on health care expenses. Debate has centered on comparing the cost and benefits of available contrast materials with their relative toxicity. Researchers have rapidly developed technological improvements, and the combination of dynamic changes in market behavior and the high cost of imaging technology in health care expenses has initiated much discussion about the types of contrast materials and their relative benefits for patients.

Ionic and nonionic contrast material

Studies have shown that blood clot formation occurs in angiographic syringes that contain nonionic contrast material. When these agents interact and coagulate blood, practitioners should remember that low osmolar nonionic contrast media exert less of an anticoagulant effect than ionic contrast media do, because the ionic contrast media interact with the hemostatic system on different levels and inhibit fibrin monomer polymerization by binding with and inactivating the protein necessary for coagulation. Ionic contrast media can also hinder the ability of thrombin to activate platelets. Nonionic agents do not affect the system in this manner. Other studies suggest that the use of ionic contrast media may be linked to reduce thrombus formation, with fewer closures of acute vessels and marked reduction in platelet deposits and thrombi during angioplasty procedures.

Barium sulfate

As a negative diamagnetic contrast agent, barium sulfate causes a loss of signal in the bowel because of 1) the predilection of barium to replace the water protons and 2) the magnetic capacity attributed to the barium particles. The results of current testing of conventional barium sulfate suspension at 60% wt/wt are encouraging. Loss of signal is greater in higher concentrations of the barium sulfate contrast agent with 170% to 220% wt/vl suspensions than in the original barium suspension. Although the loss of signal in the barium sulfate suspensions is not comparable to the loss of signal in superparamagnetic iron oxide agents, the barium suspensions are more readily available for practitioners and are usually less expensive than other contrast agents.

Water-soluble contrast agents

Water-soluble contrast agents may be preferable in studies of certain organs, such as the small bowel. Although ionic contrast agents are usually used in comparable studies, nonionic agents can be considered viable alternatives in particular circumstances when barium sulfate is contraindicated. Any inclusion of a water-soluble contrast agent should be properly documented, although such decisions should be made after radiographic quality and other clinical findings have been studied. A diagnosis of obstruction may be confirmed by radiologic findings. Practitioners should identify any fistulae or abnormal passageways from hollow organs to other hollow organs or to the surface of the skin, any obstructions in patients who have been treated with laparotomy, and any problems in the surgical section of the abdominal wall, as these conditions have not been noted in patients with negative results from previous examinations with contrast. Most patients can tolerate nonionic water-soluble follow-through examinations, which provide accurate diagnoses of any obstruction or fistula.

<u>Air as a contrast agent</u>

Air can also be used as a contrast agent in certain studies, although the use of air is not as common as the use of a liquid dye. During a study aimed at comparing air and liquid as contrast agents in the diagnosis and reduction of intussusception, or at drawing a length of intestine into an adjacent portion to produce obstruction, practitioners discovered that air enemas could be considered effective contrast agents for more than half of the patients included in the study. These results show that air is as effective a contrast agent as liquid contrast material. When air was used for fluoroscopic or x-ray viewing of opaque internal structures, the imaging times were shorter when practitioners had experience with using air as a contrast agent. Air is not always the preferred method, however, and its use should be thoroughly studied before it is implemented.

Administration routes

<u>IV administration</u>

Practitioners may choose to administer contrast materials intravenously as a bolus injection or as a continuous infusion. IV administration is acceptable for ionic or nonionic contrast agents. Butterfly needles are preferable for direct IV injections because they allow the practitioner to change large syringes more easily. For an angiocatheter IV, a 20- or 22-gauge needle should be used, and the practitioner should be experienced enough to know how much force is necessary to slide the plastic catheter over the metal stylet.

Required materials: For some CT examinations, an IV line must be inserted before testing so that the contrast agent can be administered. Before the test begins, the practitioner should gather the proper materials for administering the IV. Those materials include absorbent disposable sheets or towels; alcohol wipes for preparing the arm; a tourniquet; angiocatheter or butterfly needles; IV tubing, such as Smart Set; a 30-cc syringe filled with 30 cc of normal saline; several pieces of gauze cut into 4-in or 2-in squares; and 4 pieces of tape precut into 4-in (10-cm) strips and conveniently located at the table or stretcher. Rubber gloves should be worn at all times.

Preparation of IV tubing: Practitioners can attach to the intravenous tubing both a syringe for administering the contrast agent and a syringe for administering the saline flush. The Smart Set complements dynamic contrast injections for various tests and has one-way valves that allow the practitioner to alternate between the contrast injection and the saline flush, thereby allowing a continuous bolus with no gaps. With experience, the practitioner can also determine whether the patient has experienced any negative reactions to the injection. The practitioner should verify that no large air bubbles exist in the saline line when filling the tubing. Any off-the-shelf IV tubing should be clamped so that the saline does not drip. Most Smart Set devices have valves that are usually in a closed position.

Preparation of patient: The practitioner should introduce himself or herself to the patient before preparing the IV injection. The practitioner should ask whether the patient has previously experienced an IV injection and whether the patient would like to discuss any complications or concerns. The practitioner may educate the patient at this time about what will be done and about the purpose for the IV in relation to the CT scan. Patients who are familiar with the process involved in placing an IV may have a preferred location, such as the outer arm or hand. The patient can direct the practitioner to this area, although the antecubital fossa should be considered the default location because of the large, easily accessible antecubital vein.

Preparation of the arm: The tourniquet should be placed high on the upper arm and should be tight enough so that the skin is noticeably indented but not so tight as to cause the patient any undue discomfort. The patient may need to squeeze his or her hand so that the veins are engorged, at which point the practitioner can locate the appropriate distended subcutaneous vein. Some patients' arms will not allow for visual location of a vein; therefore, practitioners may need to palpate the arm to find an appropriate vein or to cover the arm with warm towels to assist in peripheral vasodilation. If no veins are visibly or manually located, the practitioner should release the tourniquet and reapply it to the forearm. If no veins are found in one arm, the practitioner should consider trying the other arm. The area around the selected vein should be cleaned and disinfected with alcohol wipes. Hirsute areas will need to be shaved clear before they are cleaned.

Puncturing the skin: One hand should provide counter-tension against the skin while the other hand pulls the skin distally toward the wrist in the direction opposite the needle. The counter-tension should not be strong enough to compress inflow to the vein. The angiocatheter should be advanced through the skin over the top of the vein or adjacent to the vein with a quick, jabbing motion to minimize any discomfort to the patient. The angiocatheter can then be advanced into the vein, and the practitioner should look for blood at the angiocatheter hub for verification that the angiocatheter has entered the vein successfully. For unsuccessful entrances, the practitioner should slowly pull back on the angiocatheter without fully removing it from the patient and then reattempt entry. If no blood appears in the angiocatheter hub, the practitioner should release the tourniquet, remove the needle, cover the area with gauze and tape, and try the other arm.

Oral contrast materials

Oral contrast agents depict different portions of the organ or tissues being studied, because low concentrations of paramagnetic dye can cause a reduction in T1 relaxation time, whereas high concentrations can cause T2 shortening similar to that seen with superparamagnetic iron oxide in decreasing the signal. Buffering is necessary for oral contrast because the Gd-DTPA chelates are unstable at low pH levels in the stomach.

Rectal administration

Although CT scans of differing parts of the body require various preparations, the contrast material selected for the study also has a great bearing on how the agent is introduced into the body. CT studies and scans of the gastrointestinal (GI) tract or cavities require rectal insertion of contrast material, whereas this process would be unnecessary for spinal CT.

Intrathecal administration

Intrathecal injection of contrast material requires that the contrast agent be introduced at a particular point under the arachnoid membrane of the brain or spinal cord.

Catheter administration

Catheters, or tubular medical devices, can be inserted into canals, passageways, vessels, or body cavities so that injection or removal of fluids can be completed and the passage can remain open during the examination. The practitioner is responsible for selecting the most appropriate method and the correct dosage of contrast material.

Special considerations

Allergies

Before the introduction of dye, practitioners should determine whether the patient has any medication allergies; during the procedure, practitioners should monitor the patient's vital signs closely.

Effect on patient

Before administering any contrast material to a patient, the practitioner should verify that the dye has been warmed to body temperature and that the dosage is appropriate for the test and the patient. Adults generally require a dosage of 150 to 250 mL, whereas children may require only 1 to 3 mL/kg. Spiral CT does not require the general dosage, and any overdosage can be life-threatening because the contrast material may compromise the pulmonary or cardiovascular systems. Practitioners should administer the contrast materials by rapid infusion or bolus injection and should be trained to recognize and respond to the patient's reaction to the dye, because reactions are unpredictable. Six to 100 of every million patients will experience a fatal reaction to contrast material. Because contrast material does not bind to serum protein or plasma, it cannot be dialyzed.

Excretion of contrast material

Although the expected biologic half-life of contrast materials ranges from 10 to 90 minutes, practitioners should inform patients that 90% of the contrast material will be excreted within 24 hours of injection and that the peak urine concentration of the dye will occur within 2 hours of administration. The main excretion route for any contrast material is through the kidneys, although the body can excrete the dye through the liver. Thus, patients with poor renal function are more likely to excrete the dye through the small intestine or the gallbladder. Excretions that occur during nursing of infants do not change the contrast material.

High- and low-osmolality contrast media

Osmolality is the number of particles of contrast material in any measured kilogram of water. This measure is used during the consideration of which contrast material is preferable for a particular patient and for the specific CT scan. The standard ionic contrast agent is a high-osmolality contrast medium (HOCM), which can contain 1200 to 2500 mOsm/kg water, a level 4 to 8 times the osmolality of blood, which is only 300 mOsm/kg water. HOCM is believed to be more toxic than low-osmolality contrast medium (LOCM), which is a nonionic contrast material. LOCM has an osmolality of 600 to 800 mOsm/kg water, a level only 2 to 3 times higher than that of blood. Practitioners should be mindful of which level of contrast agent has been selected.

Image resolution

Practitioners anticipate that the effects of contrast material will be noticeable during analysis because the contrast material augments the contrast resolution by an increased photoelectric effect. Any discernable contrast improvement can be directly correlated to the degree of iodine concentration in the contrast dye because the atomic number of iodine is 53 (Z:53). Peak iodine blood concentration is observed in patients within 2 minutes after the intravenous (IV) injection. At this point, the biologic half-life of the iodinated contrast material in the vascular compartment is approximately 20 minutes. The iodinated contrast material is then transferred from the vascular compartment to the extravascular compartment within 10 minutes so that the equilibrium is followed by a measured decrease in both compartments. Although severely impaired renal function results in poor contrast resolution and prolonged plasma levels, renal accumulation occurs within 1 minute, and the maximum contrast is evident within 5 to 15 minutes.

Adverse reactions

Not all patients respond to contrast agents in the same way or even in safe ways. Patients may have an adverse reaction to the nonionic iodine used during contrast-enhanced CT. Under these circumstances, practitioners should verify that the patient's vital signs are carefully monitored. For some patients, the response to contrast agents involves a negative change in the pulse rate, in the systolic and diastolic arterial blood pressure, and in the arterial blood oxygen saturation level.

Physical responses can be minor, intermediate, or severe. Nausea and pharyngeal discomfort are the most common symptoms reported by patients who experience negative reactions, although some patients have also exhibited prolonged hypotension, transient hypotension or hypertension, facial edema, and urticaria defined by raised patches of skin or mucous membranes and serious itching, sometimes with no obvious clinical symptoms. The contrast material may cause acute kidney failure in some patients, although the risk of this occurrence is higher for patients with certain pre-existing conditions. Diabetic patients may require an adjustment in medication or fluid intake so that any potential problems can be minimized during and after the procedure. All patients should drink plenty of fluids after the procedure to flush out the contrast dye. Although newer types of contrast agents are being developed to minimize possible allergic reactions, each patient should discuss any potential changes in medication before testing.

Radiation Safety and Dosimetry

Technical factors affecting patient dose

KVp and keV

High-energy electrons collide with tungsten at the end of an x-ray tube, which generates the x-rays used in medical analysis. Once the electrons are boiled off a heated wire, they are generated at the filament of the x-ray tube and receive kinetic energy because of the combination of the filament and the tungsten target. A voltage of 100,000 volts (100 kilovoltage, or kVp) is and applied to the x-ray tube. The electrons hit the tungsten with an energy level of 100 keV and can produce x-rays that are between 0 and 100 keV. Because low-energy x-rays cannot leave the x-ray tube, the resultant energy of the x-ray encompasses only 10 keV to 100 keV. Higher x-ray energy measurements indicate the degree to which the radiation penetrates tissue; thus, higher kVp measurements indicate a more intense x-ray beam.

Effect of kVp: The kVp of any test determines the energy of the x-rays, whereas the tube voltage affects the quantity of the x-rays generated. The machine can produce only a certain quantity of x-rays for any given tube voltage, and this quantity is based on the milliamps (mA) of energy currents moving through the x-ray tube. The image quality is determined by the number of x-rays that reach the film, whereas the image contrast is determined by the difference between the photons that pass through different body parts during the test. The kVp values are higher when a higher concentration of photons passes through body parts. Practitioners strive to maintain a low mA with a high kVp so that the image will have good quality and the patient will not be exposed to excessive amounts of radiation.

mAs

The current of energy expended through an x-ray tube once that tube is energized is measured in milliampere-seconds (mAs). X-ray machines operate at a particular kilovoltage potential, which is proportional to the radiation output, and the particular exposure is described by mAs. The patient radiation dose for CT is usually higher than that for radiography or fluoroscopy: the patient radiation dose during radiography is about 5 mAs or 100 mrad per examination, whereas the patient radiation dose for CT is about 50 mAs or 5000 mrad per examination. Fluoroscopy radiation dosages can range from 1000 to 100,000 mrad per examination at about 4000 mrad/min. The patient radiation dosage during CT is inversely proportional to pitch but is rather independent of collimation, or parallel entry rays. Higher pitch results in lower patient radiation dosage during any given collimation.

Pitch

Pitch in CT is calculated as the movement of the patient couch that occurs per rotation divided by the slice thickness. A contiguous spiral has 1 pitch and measures 10 mm/10 mm, whereas an extended spiral has 2 pitch and measures 20 mm/10 mm and an overlapping spiral has 1/2 pitch with a 5 mm/10 mm measurement. As pitch is lowered, z-axis resolution improves, and a combination of low pitch and narrow collimation provides better z-axis resolution than that provided by the combination of low pitch and wide collimation. However, lung nodules and other high-contrast, thin-slice examinations are best represented by low pitch and narrow collimation. When pitch measurements exceed 1, loss of the z-axis resolution can be limited only by the use of 180 interpolation. The z-axis or longitudinal coverage comprises couch velocity (mm/s) and image time (s).

Patient dose and pitch: The data from the CT imager are collected continuously but not from a transverse plane. Patient dose is reduced when the pitch of the spiral CT is increased as the patient dose is approximated to be proportional to 1/pitch. The slice thickness of the study, when divided by the couch movement, is proportional to the patient dose, and most practitioners believe that any pitch higher than 2 would be excessive and not conducive to a representative CT or any clinical examination. The adjusted couch speed, measured in mm/s, should not exceed either 10 mm/s or the slice thickness of the study so that the best compromise can be obtained between image volume and image quality. More anatomy is covered during an examination that involves a larger measurement of pitch.

Collimation

Collimation is used in CT when useful x-ray beams are restricted to the anatomical area being studied so that the patient dose can be reduced and the image contrast of the area can be improved. CT involves 2 types of collimators: pre-patient and post-patient. Pre-patient collimators are positioned near the x-ray source and control the patient dose while determining the patient profile. Patient dose increases, causing a subsequent rounding of the dose profile, when the pre-patient collimator is narrowed. Post-patient collimators determine the slice thickness used in CT, and the dose profile is configured as the plot of dose measured across the slice thickness. The ideal dose profile has a more defined, boxy shape, whereas the actual dose profile is a rounded, hill-like shape.

Radiation protection

During CT, the patient radiation dose can be almost uniform throughout the body, in contrast to the dose delivered by radiography or fluoroscopy, which is at its maximum at the entrance areas. Spiral CT often involves lesser doses of radiation because the images overlap, although they can be reconstructed with no overlapping scans. The patient radiation dose administered during CT is generally higher when the practitioner requisitions thinner slices or slices that overlap. The approximate tissue dose for a newborn's head is 4100 mrad, whereas the dosage for an adult's head is 3700 mrad because of the complexity and density of the organ. The abdomen would require an approximate patient dose of 2000 mrad for a newborn but only 1100 for an adult. The patient dose can be reduced in any x-ray imaging but at the expense of the image noise.

Shielding

Because patients are exposed to radiation during CT scanning, they must be shielded against any harmful exposure for their own protection. The shielding itself involves a material that will absorb the ionizing radiation associated with the type of test, and this protection against radiation can be extended to the patient, to medical personnel, and to members of the general public. The radiation exposure for any particular area is shaped like a figure eight; the lowest area radiation exposures are in the plane of the gantry and outside the patient aperture. The highest area radiation exposures occur near the patient and can be classified as the result of scatter radiation produced in the patient.

Personnel protection: Although radiation exposure is a concern, medical personnel can be in the same room as the CT scanner with limited effects from the radiation when they use basic shielding. The area radiation exposure from the scan plane encompasses approximately 1 mR/scan, and CT technologists can remain in the test area if they are adequately clothed in protective apparel. Whenever practitioners or other medical personnel must remain in the room, they must wear a radiation monitor no lower than at collar level above the protective apron so that levels of radiation can be checked throughout the test. All CT technologists should adhere to the practice of As Low As Reasonably Achievable (ALARA) in minimizing time spent in the area, maximizing the distance from the testing center, and using shielding at all times.

Measuring radiation exposure to personnel: All medical personnel or practitioners should maintain personal dosimetry awareness by wearing a badge and a ring during radiography and other fluoroscopic procedures, as defined by the health care organization. The badges measure exposure to the entire body, whereas the rings can more definitively measure the exposure to the extremities. The badges and rings should be stored in a safe, clean area, and practitioners should wear the most current badge that has been specifically designed for each member. The badge should be worn outside the lead apron around the middle of the body. The extremity ring should be worn beneath leaded gloves whenever the practitioner holds any items related to the study.

Exposure times for personnel: Occasionally, practitioners will be required to hold patients during CT scanning. Under such circumstances, the practitioner should consider decreasing the exposure time and should use proper radiographic exposure techniques during the examination so as to reduce the need to repeat any exposures or to refocus the tests. Holding patients during scanning should the last option for completing the scan. Personnel who hold the patient should be alternated for each test so that no one person endures prolonged radiation exposure. Patients undergoing CT testing will be anesthetized, mechanically restrained, or tranquilized during the test; however, if practitioners must physically hold the patient, they should wear lead gloves during the procedure.

Procedures for protection: Only essential personnel should be in the room during the test, and the distance from the radiation to the exposed practitioner should be increased. Any practitioner who is holding a patient should be as far from the beam as possible. During the radiographic exposure, no one is allowed outside the control booth or past the yellow safety line, which shows the personnel the location of scatter radiation exposure. The walls of the CT room should be leaded, and practitioners should remain behind the control panel shield during testing for protection against scatter radiation. The x-ray beams should never be pointed directly at the shields, and all practitioners should wear lead aprons, lead gloves, and thyroid shields. No medical personnel should ever be in the direct path of the radiographic beam. Lead-impregnated glasses should be worn when necessary so that eye exposure to tube leakage and scatter radiation can be reduced.

Scatter radiation

Once x-ray beams interact with matter, such as tissues, organs, protective clothing, and each other, those beams change direction. Classic scattering is the changing of the direction of the x-ray beams without a subsequent loss of energy; it is defined as coherent, Rayleigh, or Thompson scattering. Compton scattering is the ionization and x-ray scattering that result from the interaction between the x-ray and a loosely bound outer-shell electron, also known as a Compton electron, which is emitted from the outer shell of the atom in response to x-ray scattering. Scatter radiation can reduce contrast and produce less contrast resolution in the image, whereas larger pre-patient and post-patient collimation produces more scatter radiation.

Dosimetry

Dosimetry is the theory and application of various techniques and principles used by CT technologists and other practitioners to measure and record the radiation dose to the patient participating in the CT examination. This study can also be extended to medical personnel in the same area during CT scanning and other comparable tests. Studies measure the quantitative facets of the CT to determine the spatial and temporal radiation exposure associated with a particular test at a particular dose for a particular patient. The radiation is measured by a dosimeter, which can be adjusted to detect and define the exposure of the instrument and subsequent patients or practitioners to any ionizing radiation in the area.

CTDI and MSAD

CT examinations that specify a patient dose will usually include an average value for the dose distribution, and the patient dose used in CT examinations can be measured with a pencil ionization chamber. The dose profile can be the most helpful guide in determining and identifying the patient dose, and patient doses in CT are described by the CT dose index (CTDI). The CTDI must be comparable in some way to the multiple-scan average dose (MSAD) because the CTDI can equal the MSAD only if the slice thickness of the test equals the couch incrementation. If the slice thickness is not equivalent to the couch incrementation, then the MSAD must be equal to the CTDI multiplied by the couch incrementation.

Limitations

CTDI and MSAD assist in characterizing and differentiating physical dose quantities between programs and systems that work with radiation exposure. Practitioners incorporate CTDI and MSAD in evaluating the exposure of patients to radiation during CT, because these measures are useful in determining the absorbed doses of radiation being examined. However, CTDI and MSAD cannot demonstrate the biological sensitivity of the organs being imaged with CT, nor can they accurately describe the radiogenic risk faced by patients and practitioners. Other methods of measurement, such as the dose on the axis of rotation, also cannot provide accurate determinations of the radiogenic risk for patients; thus, when declaring an acceptable dose limit, practitioners should consider other regions of study so that the image created during the CT will be conducive to study and the patient and practitioner can avoid any unnecessarily high risks of exposure.

Effective dose

As an alternative method of determining the dose quantity, practitioners can use the effective dose measurement, which considers the dose required for the particular organ being studied and the tissue-weighting factors, which generally range from .01 to .20. A rough estimate of the average effective dose requirement for the head would be .0025 mSv/mGy*cm, whereas the dose for the trunk would be .0175 mSv/mGy*cm.

CTDI and MSAD depend on the particular scan or rotation being implemented, whereas the dose depends on the kVp, mAs, and slice collimation. The effective dose measurement is determined for each examination, and the dose is based on patient-related factors such as the integral dose, the body region being studied, and patient size.

Pediatric dose reduction

Practitioners are reluctant to complete CT examinations on pediatric patients because of uncertainty about the dose that will facilitate an image useful for studying a particular body part. Pediatric patients cannot withstand the same amount of radiation as adult patients, and this limitation must be accounted for in determining the dosage. Ongoing research is aimed at developing an acceptable method of determining pediatric dose reduction as it relates to image quality. Practitioners and other medical personnel have used mathematical formulas and digital in-painting techniques to create artificial body parts with lesions and other growths that could be as significant as 6 mm. Through simulation, researchers can compare doses with image quality without endangering pediatric patients unnecessarily.

Imaging Procedures

Type of Study

CT of the head

Need IV contrast agents

CT scans of the head are necessary for various conditions or circumstances leading to the patient's arrival at an emergency facility. When a patient loses consciousness, is discovered in a prone position on the floor with no obvious reason for falling, experiences intensely painful headaches, or experiences seizures for the first time, the practitioner should consider this a nontrauma incident with no need for IV contrast agents. If the patient is known to have brain pathology and experiences a follow-up condition, the practitioner should consider this a nontrauma incident and request IV contrast agents. If the patient has experienced any kind of penetration, head trauma with loss of consciousness, lacerations, raccoon eyes, unequal or abnormal pupils, hemotympanum, depressed skull, or cephalhematoma, the practitioner should consider this a trauma incident with no need for IV contrast agents.

Bones of the skull

The skull itself consists of 12 bones fused together in conjunction. These bones are the orbital plate of frontal bones located at the eyebrows; the benign hyperostosis frontalis at the top of the forehead; the groove for the posterior division of the middle meningeal artery above and behind the ear; the anterior clinoid process just below the temple; the posterior clinoid process just above the ear; the sphenoid sinus at the front of the ear; the planum sphenoidale at the corner of the eye; the petrous pyramid at the top of the spine; the external auditory canal to the front of the spine top; the lambdoidal suture at the back of the head; the hypophyseal fossa within the ear; and the superimposed coronal suture and inner table vascular grooves at the middle of the skull.

Skull base

The skull base comprises the anterior cranial fossa, the middle fossa, and the posterior cranial fossa with each portion in its approximate degree of the skull, starting from the front and moving toward the back. The anterior cranial fossa consists of the frontal sinuses and the lesser sphenoidal wings, which compose the orbital plate of the frontal bone and the crista galli, with the cribriform plate and planum sphenoidale existing between. As the superior surface of the body of the sphenoid bone, the planum sphenoidale is a continuous structure with the tuberculum sellae or the front surface of the hypophyseal fossa, also called the pituitary, which serves as a middle cranial fossa structure.

Middle cranial fossa

The middle cranial fossa contains the hypophyseal fossa that is bracketed by the back of the tuberculum and the anterior clinoid processes, the bottom of the hypophyseal fossa, and the front of the dorsum sellae and associated posterior clinoids. The bottom of the middle cranial fossa includes the foramen spinosum, the foramen ovale, the foramen rotundum, which contains the maxillary nerve, and the foramen lacerum, which acts as a false foramen as it is covered by thin fibrous tissue. The back part is the greater sphenoidal wing, whereas the middle meningeal artery reaches across the inner table of the base from front to back. The rest of the lateral wall of the middle fossa consists of the squamosal portion of the temporal bone, which includes the mastoid process and air cells and the external auditory canal. The petrous pyramid includes the tympanic membrane, the middle ear bones, the inner ear bones, and the cochlea.

Posterior cranial fossa

At the back, the posterior cranial fossa is bracketed by the dorsum sellae continuously joined to the clivus, the back of the petrous pyramid, alongside the parietal bones, and at the back of the occipital bone. As the largest opening of the skull and located at the occipital bone, the foramen magnum allows a connection between the brain and the medulla oblongata or spinal cord, also called the spinal medulla. The basion and opisthion form the midsagittal plane of the anterior arc of the foramen magnum, with the basion acting as the fundamentally important landmark in determining the occipital-atlantal relationship. The jugular foramen is bilateral to the foramen magnum and transmits the jugular vein, which serves as the anterior extension of the superior sagittal sinus as it continues toward the transverse and sigmoid sinuses. These sinuses exhibit inner table grooves that may be visible on regular CT scans.

Constant openings in the fossae: The anterior, middle, and posterior cranial fossae have constant openings within the bone structures. The anterior cranial fossa has its constant opening in the cribriform plate foramina, whereas the posterior cranial fossa has constant openings in more than one location. Those constant openings include the foramen magnum, the internal auditory meatus, the jugular foramen, and the hypoglossal canal. The middle cranial fossa, on the other hand, contains most of the constant openings within the bone structure. There are constant openings in the optic canal, the superior orbital fissure, the foramen spinosum, the foramen ovale, the foramen rotundum, the foramen lacerum, and the hiatus for the greater and lesser petrosal nerves in the middle cranial fossa. These constant openings allow for movement and transference of fluid between the fossae.

Pituitary gland

Referred to as the master gland, the pituitary gland controls the functions of other endocrine glands. Located at the base of the brain, the pituitary gland is the size of a pea and is attached by nerve fibers to the hypothalamus, the part of the brain affecting the pituitary gland. The gland itself consists of anterior, intermediate, and posterior lobes, each of which produces certain hormones. The anterior lobe produces growth hormone; prolactin, which stimulates milk production in women after giving birth; adrenocorticotropic hormone (ACTH), which stimulates the adrenal glands; thyroid-stimulating hormone (TSH); follicle-stimulating hormone (FSH), which stimulates ovaries or testes; and luteinizing hormone (LH), which stimulates ovaries or testes. The intermediate lobe produces melanocyte-stimulating hormone, which controls skin pigmentation. The posterior lobe produces antidiuretic hormone (ADH), which increases water absorption by the kidneys, and oxytocin, which contracts the uterus during childbirth.

Orbits

CT scanning allows evaluation of the orbits. Bone algorithms are used to evaluate the orbital walls for trauma; soft-tissue algorithms are used to provide contrast for detecting inflammatory or neoplastic processes.

Paranasal sinuses

CT scanning assists practitioners in evaluating the inflammatory and neoplastic processes of the paranasal sinuses. The examination is normally performed by using a bone algorithm to accentuate the osseous structures without the need for a contrast dye.

Temporal bones

For the evaluation of temporal bones with axial and coronal images, CT scans offer thin-section (approximately 1 mm) collimations so that practitioners can review the structures of the inner and middle ear. This type of scanning allows the evaluation of various auditory structures for congenital malformations; such evaluations are necessary when ear implants are being considered. CT is preferable to other imaging methods for detecting acute trauma or a temporal bone fracture.

Maxillofacial region

The maxillofacial region consists of the upper jaw or face, with particular emphasis on the maxilla, the jaw that is fused to the cranium and is referred to as the upper jaw or the upper jawbone. Practitioners who specialize in oral and maxillofacial surgery complete at least 5 years of basic medical studies before completing 4 years of more-specialized medical and dental training. Maxillofacial studies involve extensive research into the diagnosis and treatment of various diseases that affect the mouth, teeth, face, and neck, including oral and dentoalveolar surgery for impacted and buried teeth or cysts; preprosthetic surgery for bone augmentation; placement of dental implants to replace missing teeth or retain facial prostheses; orthognathic surgery for dentofacial deformities; reconstructive and aesthetic surgery; and procedures for correcting temporomandibular joint disorder (TMJD), facial trauma, tumors, cleft lip and palate, and congenital craniofacial deformities.

Purpose of the maxillae: The maxillae are the largest bones of the face, excluding the mandible; their union forms the upper jaw in its entirety. The maxillae hold the upper teeth and connect to the zygomatic bones, or cheek bones, at the right and left sides of the face. The sections of the maxillae form the boundaries of the 3 cavities of the upper jaw: the roof of the mouth, the floor and lateral wall of the nose, and the floor of the orbit. Each bone of the maxillae consists of the body of the maxilla, as well as the zygomatic process, the frontal process, the alveolar process, and the palatine process. The maxillae consist of nine bones: the frontal and ethmoid bones of the cranium, the nasal bone, the zygomatic bone, the lacrimal bone, the inferior nasal concha, the palatine bone, and both vomer articulations. The maxilla forms part of the anterior and middle fossae, as well as the interior orbital and pterygomaxillary fissures. The maxilla will sometimes articulate with the lateral pterygoid plate of the sphenoid bone or with the orbital surface.

Maxillofacial surgeons: Maxillofacial surgery is a very specialized branch of medicine, but maxillofacial surgeons can work alongside other specialists in repairing damage or trauma, or in treating facial deformities or abnormalities. These other specialists include dentists, orthodontists, pathologists, oncologists, restorative dentists, radiologists, plastic surgeons, ENT surgeons, neurosurgeons, and other professionals who correct deformities of the maxillae. Maxillofacial surgery is focused enough that specialization and cooperation are required for effective service.

Temporomandibular joints

The temporomandibular joints (TMJs) are 2 matching joints on each side of the head below and in front of the ears; they connect the lower jaw to the skull. Although the abbreviation TMJ literally describes the joint, it can also be used to identify the symptoms or disorders experienced by most patients with facial pain or discomfort originating at the lower jaw. These problems might include jaw pain, popping sounds upon extending the jaw, headaches, earaches, toothaches, inability to extend the mouth fully, and other related facial pains. The problems caused by TMJ disorders result from physical or emotional stress placed upon the structures surrounding the jaw: muscles, face, neck, teeth, cartilage disc at the joint, nearby ligaments, blood vessels, and nerves.

TMJ disorders: Patients who grind their teeth may experience TMJ disorders; this grinding can be unconscious during sleep or conscious in response to daily stress. The teeth are slid across each other, usually with a sideways, back-and-forth motion, and this activity can disrupt the sleep of others and can also wear down the patient's teeth over time. The clenching of the jaw clamps the bottom and top teeth together with greater emphasis on the back teeth, and the stressful force of the clenching puts pressure on the muscles, tissues, and other structures that make up and surround the jaw. Poor posture, such as that usually associated with long hours spent working at a computer, can place unnecessary strain on the face and neck. In addition, poor diet, arthritis, lack of sleep, fractures, dislocations, and structural problems can contribute to the pain of TMJ disorders.

Brain

Computed tomography (CT) was first used to produce images of the brain, and this has been its most traditional use in radiological examinations since its implementation. CT of the brain is the method preferred by practitioners who must treat patients who have experienced acute head trauma and those who present with focal neurological deficits that may be the result of an acute intracranial hemorrhage. This type of neuroimaging allows practitioners to exploit the sensitivity of CT scanning to rule out intracranial hemorrhaging and acute ischemic stroke. CT scans are less accurate than MRI tests in detecting early ischemic strokes, intracranial metastatic disease, and white matter degenerative changes, but the CT scan provides a basis for further analysis and can be used in emergency circumstances, for example, to detect the type of damage suffered during head trauma.

Practitioners should request that patients remove hair accessories or partial dental plates, because these items may block the images of brain tissue. The patient lies on the examination table with the head on a support so that it may be secured during the test. The face is not covered, although patients will be unable to see outside the machine during testing. An x-ray beam is sent by the scanner to move from one side of the brain to the other, and the machine rotates 1 degree before sending another x-ray beam across the brain. The process is usually repeated over a range of 180 degrees; the machine is then moved to begin the same process at as many as 7 angles or planes. Patients hear a clicking sound while the scanning device moves around the head. CT scanning of the brain usually lasts less than 60 minutes.

Images of the brain: The communication pathway for the flow of cerebrospinal fluid (CSF) from the aqueduct and central canal of the medulla is at the level of the middle-posterior cranial fossae or the fourth ventricle, between the pons and the cerebellum. The basilar artery sits in front of the pons, is formed by the intersection of 2 vertebral arteries, and begins the 2 posterior cerebral arteries. The petrous pyramids on an axial image show the frontal and temporal lobes, along with the cerebellum. The middle cerebral artery comes from part of the internal carotid artery in the Sylvian fissure. The brain stem comprises the pons, the medulla, and the mesencephalon and is surrounded by the perimesencephalic cistern. The suprasellar cistern is five-pointed and contains the pituitary gland and most of the internal carotid artery. The interpeduncular fossa is triangular in shape, and the fourth and third ventricles are connected by the aqueduct and extend through the midbrain.

Axial images of the anterior and posterior parts of the third ventricle can show the confluence of sinuses and the superior vermes of the cerebellum. Higher slices can also show the anterior horn of the lateral ventricle, the caudate head, the anterior limb of the internal capsule, the lentiform nucleus, the external capsule, the insular cortex, and the straight sinus. The pineal gland is surrounded by the superior cerebellar cistern, and the occipital lobes are visible above the tentorium and are separated by the posterior interhemispheric fissure. With higher levels of radiation, the CT scan can show the body of the third ventricle, the posterior horn of the lateral ventricle, and the vein of Galen. The anterior portion of the bodies of the lateral ventricles is separated at the roof of the third ventricle by the septum pellucidum, and the posterior horns are separated by the splenium of the corpus callosum.

The concave nature of the anterior horn of the lateral ventricle is at the olive-shaped caudate head or nucleus. The corpus callosum separates the bodies of the lateral ventricles from the choroids plexus. The corpus callosum is broader at the top of the bodies of the lateral ventricles than at the more caudal levels, although the straight sinus drains into the posterior part of the sagittal sinus. The cerebral sulci and gyri, as well as the falx, become visible throughout the length of the interhemispheric fissure. The gray-white interface of the gyri becomes clearly visible near the vortex of the central hemispheres, and the precentral sulcus and gyrus, the central sulcus, and the postcentral sulcus and gyrus are identifiable. The sagittal sinus within the interhemispheric fissure also becomes evident at that level. Physiological dural calcifications may be present on the sagittal sinus, which is usually visible on the superior-most image of the brain.

Cranium

Intracranial bleeding: Practitioners have used CT scans to identify normal and abnormal structures after intracranial bleeding. CT scans allow for fast and accurate diagnosis of intracranial bleeding and have become favored over cerebral angiography in acute trauma facilities. Patients with multiple injuries are handled differently than patients with only head injuries, although patients with head injuries that cause intracranial bleeding may demonstrate intracranial abnormalities almost immediately after the injury or during the following few days. CT scans allow practitioners to monitor this potential development and to work with patients to minimize intracranial bleeding and edema. CT is painless and can be indispensable to practitioners who believe, as the result of CT findings, that the patient requires immediate medical attention.

Cleidocranial dysplasia: Previously diagnosed by plain x-rays of the cranium and chest, cleidocranial dysplasia (CCD) is an autosomal dominant disorder that is associated with the absence or hypoplasia of the clavicles, malalignment of the teeth, and an open fontanelle. A clear view of the open fontanelle is provided by 3D CT; radiographs of the skull do not demonstrate this structure as conclusively. Practitioners have used 3D CT to diagnose CCD in older children, who may have presented with hypertelorism, a broad and flat nasal bridge, an open anterior fontanelle, and a bell-shaped thorax as seen on a CT scan of the chest, and with narrowed upper portions or complete absence of both clavicles and Wormian bones in the cranium. The open fontanelle is not always clearly visualized in older children with CCD unless 3D CT is used, because these older children have more mineralization in the cranium and a thicker calvarial bone.

Although practitioners can reconstruct a transverse planar image at any position along the patient's axis, difficulty arises during the interpolation of spiral CT images over the conventional CT. Interpolation allows the transverse image to be reconstructed from the spiral data before undergoing filtered back projection with a strong preference for 180° interpolation, even though most medical facilities offer both 180° and 360° interpolation. For young children with CCD, especially those who are small for their age, a useful 3D reconstruction of the cranium is more likely to be produced by spiral CT scanning with 4-mm-thick slices. The presence or absence of the open fontanelle is clearly defined by spiral CT, whereas other tests may show the open fontanelle only in the lateral view, not in the anteroposterior view.

Sclerosteosis: Also known as Van Buchem's disease, sclerosteosis occurs during early childhood and progressively involves the skull. Sclerosteosis is a rare, genetic disease with a dominant inheritance pattern. It causes craniotubular hyperostosis with symmetrical and bilateral diaphyseal cortical thickening of short and long tubular bones, and sclerosis and thickening of the mandible, the calvaria, the shoulder and pelvic girdles, and the thoracic cage. Alkaline phosphatase activity is usually normal, and no noted basal foramina encroachment of the skull is seen. CT will normally show no periosteal excrescences, and the pathologic changes in the cranium are usually defined.

Sclerosteosis is an incurable disease, but practitioners use CT in their analysis of the cranium before performing palliative surgery.

CT scans can provide practitioners with a better preoperative understanding of the corrections that need to be made. However, not all surgical options include removing a foreign body or curing an illness; instead, some may focus on providing the patient with relief of the pain or discomfort brought on by the development of the disease. Palliative surgery for sclerosteosis can remove an obstruction, relieve pain, or provide the patient with the ability to move and function normally. The surgery itself is an option for patients who experience discomfort due to sclerosteosis. Practitioners endeavor to improve the patient's quality of life with no assurances that this genetic disease will be cured or that life will be prolonged.

CT of the neck

Larynx

CT of the larynx became widespread in the 1970s when practitioners discovered that CT could assist in diagnosing various diseases and trauma of the larynx. MRI has become more accessible for evaluating the larynx, but CT imaging provides more detailed information about the larynx in showing potential trauma, foreign bodies, neoplasm, and other abnormalities. CT scans can isolate the site and degree of pathology in the fat and muscle of the larynx, although MRI is more sensitive in detecting pathologic involvement of the cartilage. CT is better than MRI in delineating occult fractures and dislocations. Patients who cannot remain still for long periods of time because of coughing have better success with CT than with MRI, but the radiologist is often responsible for choosing the type of study to be performed.

Benign and malignant masses: The larynx consists of the supraglottic larynx or vestibule, the laryngeal ventricle, the false cords, aryepiglottic folds, and the true cords or glottis. Specific benign masses of the larynx include laryngocele, an air- or water-filled outpouching of the laryngeal ventricle submissive to the obstruction of the laryngeal saccule and common among wind-instrument musicians; inflammatory lesions, also referred to as laryngitis, epiglottis, and croup; and papillomas, benign neoplasms usually found on the true cords with the potential for malignant transformation. Malignant neoplasms of the larynx include supraglottic squamous cell carcinoma, which could require a voice-saving supraglottic laryngectomy within certain limits, and glottic squamous cell cancer, which is confined to one vocal cord without extension and can be operable within limits. CT allows practitioners to determine the condition of the larynx and to determine whether surgery is possible.

Soft tissues of the neck

Research has focused on improving the viability of MRI for scans of the soft tissues of the neck, but MRI cannot yet provide images that are sufficient to allow practitioners to adequately examine those tissues or to determine the necessary treatment for correcting defects. CT of the soft tissues of the neck requires the use of intravenous contrast agents so that best image can be obtained. For patients with suspected inflammatory processes in the neck, CT can detect defined neck masses, potential or actual cases of head and neck cancer, and lymphoma.

Vascular

Carotid arteries: High-resolution contrast is necessary for enhanced spiral CT of the carotid artery, with a preferred scan range from the aortic arch to the circle of Willis. With a helical or spiral scan mode, the practitioner should establish scan parameters of 120 kVp with a minimum of 280 mA at one second. Collimation and slice spacing should be equal at 0.6 mm, and the patient should be instructed to perform a single breathhold with no movement during the study. The patient should not be shifted or allowed to change position during the test, and practitioners should avoid changing the table height or field of view (FOV) during the scan. A standard nonionic contrast agent may be administered at a dose of 140 mL and a rate of 3-4 mL/sec. With a standard reconstruction algorithm, the scan delay should be ROI −90 HU with FOV at 28 and window level at 400/40.

Alternative protocol for carotid arteries: High-resolution contrast is necessary for enhanced spiral CT of the carotid artery, with an alternative scan range from the aortic arch to the circle of Willis. With a helical or spiral scan mode, the practitioner should establish scan parameters of 120 kVp with a minimum of 280 mA at one second. Collimation and slice spacing should be equal at 1.25 mm, and the patient should be instructed to perform a single breathhold with no movement during the study. The patient should not be shifted or allowed to change position during the test, and practitioners should avoid changing the table height or FOV during the scan. A standard nonionic contrast agent may be administered at a dose of 140 mL and a rate of 3-4 mL/sec. With a standard reconstruction algorithm, the scan delay should be ROI −90 HU (or 15-20 seconds) with FOV at 28 and window level at 400/40.

CT of the chest

Mediastinum

The mediastinum is located between the pleural sacs of the lungs and contains all of the tissues and organs in the chest excluding the lungs and pleurae. The trachea, as shown by CT, is approximately 9 to 15 cm long and connects the lower respiratory tract to the upper respiratory tract. The trachea is classified as being in the superior and middle mediastinum. The esophagus is approximately 25 to 30 cm long and connects the lower digestive tract to the upper digestive tract; it is classified as being in the superior and posterior mediastinum. CT shows that the esophagus is behind the trachea; it receives blood from the aorta and the left gastric and inferior phrenic arteries and supplying blood to the portal venous system. The esophagus has no serosa, which makes it more susceptible to endoscopy than other organs of the digestive tract.

Lungs

CT provides practitioners with more insight into the condition of the lungs than the typical images produced by standard chest radiographs. CT of the chest can show the healthy status of normal lungs, as well as any possible abnormalities that may have gone undetected by a standard radiograph. The abnormalities evident on the CT image may be benign but could indicate the potential for a serious condition or illness. CT scans may reveal nodules in the lungs; further testing would be required to verify whether any malignancy is present. Practitioners can also verify the presence of any lesions or tumors as well as small tissue variations that would have been missed by standard radiographs.

Pulmonary arteriography: Pulmonary arteriography can show the blood vessels in the lungs (the pulmonary arteries). Once the patient has been prepared for this procedure, the practitioner will administer contrast agents. Although not all CT scans require the use of contrast material, pulmonary arteriography normally requires the use of a contrast agent because the veins and arteries are not normally visible on the x-ray. The practitioner will inject the appropriate contrast agent into one or more veins or arteries so that they can be seen on the CT image. Pulmonary arteriography can also detect clots or other blockages that may be obstructing normal blood flow through the lungs.

Scan delay for spiral CT: Practitioners have performed prospective research to determine the optimal scan delay for spiral CT in diagnosing acute pulmonary embolism. Through evaluations of easily obtained clinical parameters, practitioners have compared the image quality of a fixed scan delay with that of individualized contrast timing. Although there was no great difference between contrast times in blood pressure, heart rate, weight, body length, body surface area, or cardiac function, the contrast transit times were significantly associated with patients' age and sex. The quality of the images was not markedly different between the group assigned to a 20-second fixed scan delay and the group assigned to an individualized delay based on the transit time required for the contrast agent to move through the pulmonary circulation. The image quality was comparable for the two groups.

Heart

Right and left pulmonary veins: The right and left pulmonary veins deliver oxygen-rich blood to the left atrium, although the pulmonary veins are inferior to the pulmonary arteries. CT shows that these veins are anterior to the right pulmonary arteries in the right hilum; the left pulmonary veins are usually superior to the right.

Interventricular septum: The interventricular septum is a muscle located between the ventricles.

Coronary sinus: The coronary sinus is the large vessel that drains blood from the heart and returns it to the right atrium. CT shows that the coronary sinus travels in a groove between the left atrium and ventricle as a tributary for the great, middle, and small cardiac veins.

Tricuspid valve: The tricuspid valve is one of 4 valves in the heart. CT shows that the tricuspid valve has 3 cusps to separate the right atrium from the right ventricle.

Right ventricle: The right ventricle is the chamber of the heart that receives deoxygenated blood from the right atrium before pumping it toward the lungs so that the blood can be enriched with oxygen. The tricuspid valve separates the right ventricle and atrium. CT shows that the right ventricle is most proximal to the anterior of the thorax with well-developed thick muscles, or trabeculae carnae, and can enlarge because of blood flow resistance through the lungs.

Right atrium: The right atrium receives deoxygenated blood that returns from the body directly from the coronary sinus, the superior vena cava, and the inferior vena cava. CT can show whether there is any communication between the right and left atria, such as a patent foramen ovale, which is common among newborns. Such communication could allow emboli to originate from the venous side of the body and pass to the arterial side, thereby causing a stroke.

Left atrium: The left atrium receives oxygen-rich blood that returns from the lungs via the pulmonary veins; it pumps this blood to the left ventricle for delivery to the rest of the body. The left atrium can be affected by mitral stenosis, an obstruction of blood flow from the left atrium to the left ventricle, which causes enlargement of the atrium. CT shows the enlarged left atrium as a bulge in the posterior of the heart; this bulge can indent the esophagus.

Left ventricle: The left ventricle generates the high pressure necessary to deliver the oxygenated blood to the body. Its two-cusped mitral valve prevents backward flow into the atrium. The chordae tendineae are the strong muscles that hold the aortic valve in place. CT shows that the left ventricle is supplied by the left anterior descending coronary artery and the left circumflex artery. The left ventricle can be enlarged as the result of chronic high blood pressure.

> **Review Video: The Heart**
> Visit mometrix.com/academy and enter code: 451339

Vascular systems

As the network of blood vessels inside the body, the vascular system can be studied with cross-sectional CT images so that practitioners can observe how the flow of blood progresses in the vessels. The computer provides a detailed view of the part of the body being studied; the images are more detailed and provide more information than could be gathered from a conventional x-ray. Practitioners will normally know which vascular region is associated with the particular body part to be studied, and this focus allows the practitioners to view the area before surgery. Depending on the patient, CT may provide information about biopsies of suspected cancer, drainage of abscesses deep in the body, or removal of internal body fluids for different tests. These types of tests are minimally invasive and can usually be completed without involving surgery.

The introduction of multidetector scanners greatly affected CT scanning for vascular imaging because CTA can evaluate the arteries and vessels in multiple regions of the body, such as the brain, neck, chest, abdomen, pelvis, and extremities. Most practitioners use a 64-slice CT scanner to evaluate the coronary arteries in a process that allows diagnostic interpretation of coronary artery plaques without using an invasive procedure, as is the case with traditional coronary angiography. Unlike traditional angiography, CTA allows practitioners to evaluate the surrounding soft tissues beyond those made more opaque by the contrast agent within the blood vessel. This increased sensitivity provides a better characterization of the vessel walls and plaque development and greatly assists in individualized surgical and interventional planning.

CT of the Abdomen

CT offers practitioners views of the upper abdomen, which is located between the thorax and the pelvis. The abdomen contains such organs as the liver, stomach, and intestines. The liver comprises 4 different lobes, which occupy 4 different quadrants. As the largest organ inside the body, the liver secretes bilirubin and bile salts into the bile ducts and works as a complex navigational center for blood flow, making it the source of massive bleeding in patients who sustain blunt abdominal trauma. CT shows that the right lobe of the liver is in the upper quadrant; the left lobe is smaller and has a dissimilar blood supply and portal drainage; the caudate lobe functions with part of the right and left lobes because it receives blood from the right and left hepatic arteries; and the quadrate lobe functions with part of the left lobe because it receives blood from the left hepatic artery.

Patient preparation

Before abdominal CT scanning, patients should be informed that they will be required to lie on a special table before being moved into a body scanner, an encircling camera that looks like a large tube. That tube takes various pictures of the patient's abdomen and pelvis, using x-ray beams to create cross-sectional images of the body. Those beams are directed at thousands of points around the body as determined by the computer and the practitioner supervising the CT scan. The test usually occurs in the radiology department or in a separate CT laboratory, depending on the medical facility. The practitioner may discuss specific topics or issues with the patient during the test by using special audio equipment built into the body scanner. A conventional abdominal CT scan requires 30 to 45 minutes, whereas helical scanning generally requires less time.

Liver

The complexity of the blood flow through the liver causes it to be a delicately balanced organ susceptible to severe damage should the patient sustain blunt abdominal trauma with extensive damage to the right upper quadrant. The liver has a thin covering called Glisson's capsule of the liver; pain is produced by this covering when the liver is compromised by enlargement. When blood enters the liver through the portal vein, it originates from the blood moving through the superior mesenteric, splenic, and inferior mesenteric veins. Incoming blood also originates from the common hepatic artery, which acts as one of 3 branches extending from the celiac trunk. Middle, right, and left hepatic veins unite to create venous drainage, and these vessels work to drain blood into the inferior vena cava.

Gallbladder

The gallbladder stores bile that has been produced by the liver and releases this bile when the enzyme cholecystokinin is secreted by the duodenal cells. Palpable under the right costal margin only when it is enlarged because of inflammation or cholecystitis, gallstones, or cancer, the gallbladder is shown by CT to sit between the right and quadrate lobes of the liver and anterior to the duodenum and the transverse colon. Cholecystitis is caused when a gallstone erodes through the gallbladder wall and into the adjacent duodenum, which causes intestinal obstruction. The blood supply originates from the cystic artery, usually a branch of the right hepatic artery, and may pose concerns for practitioners performing cholecystectomy. Practitioners should also consider variations in the bile ducts of the gallbladder, which may also cause concern during surgery.

Spleen

Located in the left upper quadrant, the spleen has an upper pole that relates to the lower ribs, whereas its most inferior portion extends to L2. The tip of the spleen is usually palpable only when enlarged, as is the case with conditions such as thalassemia or leukemia. CT shows that the spleen is held in place by gastrosplenic and splenorenal ligaments and the tail of the pancreas, which is also in the splenorenal ligament of the hilum of the spleen. As a highly vascular organ, the spleen hosts cells of the reticuloendothelial system, which are responsible for producing opsonins and antibodies to fight off infection and other foreign invaders. The spleen can also be the site of severe hemorrhaging in patients who suffer sustained blunt abdominal trauma, especially to the left upper quadrant.

Pancreas

Located in the epigastrium, the pancreas is divided into 4 parts, with the head and body outside the peritoneum and important anatomical relations surrounding the organ. CT shows that the head of the pancreas is surrounded by the duodenum; the common bile duct crosses the head of the pancreas to join with the pancreatic duct at the ampulla of Vater before emptying into the descending or second part of the duodenum. The pancreatic ducts of Santorini and Wirsung drain the exocrine pancreas; the tail is located in the splenorenal ligament and enters the hilum of the spleen. The blood flow of the pancreas begins at the superior and inferior pancreaticoduodenal artery as the 2 vessels arise from the gastroduodenal artery and the superior mesenteric artery. Pancreatic cancer causes the head of the pancreas to enlarge and press against the bile duct, which causes an obstruction in bile flow and leads to clinical jaundice.

Adrenal glands

The right adrenal gland is horseshoe-shaped and is divided into the medulla and the cortex; the two parts having differing embryological origins. CT shows that the right adrenal gland is superior and medial to the kidney and that the left adrenal gland is above the right adrenal gland. The outer cortex secretes mineralocorticoids to control salt metabolism and produces glucocorticoid (cortisol) and male and female sex hormones. The adrenal medulla is the origin of chromaffin cells; it produces norepinephrine and epinephrine during normal activity and produces substantial amounts of epinephrine and norepinephrine when it is infected by pheochromocytoma, a disease that leads to hypertension and headaches. The blood flow to the adrenal glands originates from the superior, middle, and inferior suprarenal arteries.

Kidneys

The right and left kidneys are retroperitoneal, located in the posterior abdomen. The right kidney is situated 2 to 8 cm lower than the left kidney; the liver sits superior to both. Surrounded by a layer of fascia, or Gerota's renal fascia, the kidneys are divided into sections that contain the perinephric and paranephric fat that surrounds them. CT shows that the kidneys are inside a fibrous capsule that protects them from the spread of infection but is easily removed. The kidneys are complex in structure; they receive their blood supply from the renal artery, a branch of the abdominal aorta. The right renal artery travels posteriorly to the IVC toward the right kidney, and the left renal vein crosses the aorta anteriorly to reach the left kidney. The renal artery enters the capsule before dividing into segments.

Ureter: A tubular structure receiving urine from the kidneys and delivering urine to the urinary bladder, the ureter is a muscular tube approximately 25 cm long and 5 mm wide. Considered the continuation of the renal pelvis, the ureter provides peristaltic waves to push the urine to the bladder. As a retroperitoneal structure, the ureter descends into the pelvis. CT shows that the ureter is anterior to the psoas muscle and crosses the pelvic brim at the bifurcation of the common iliac artery, where it enters the bladder from a posterior and superior aspect. In the male, the ureter is lateral to the ductus deferens; in the female, the ureters are crossed anteriorly by the uterine artery before they enter the bladder.

GI tract

Stomach: Made up of the cardia, fundus, body, antrum, and pylorus, the stomach is located in the left hypogastric and epigastric regions and can extend to the pelvis when filled with food. The cardia is located at the intersection of the stomach and esophagus. The fundus is the largest portion of the stomach and can be easily visualized on CT images as a bubble. The blood supply originates from the left gastric, splenic, and common hepatic arteries, all of which are branches of the celiac plexus, and is rich with anastomoses; thus, the stomach does not suffer ischemia if a single blood supply is obstructed. The parietal cells of the fundus secrete a gastric intrinsic factor necessary for absorbing vitamin B12. Gastric ulcers can occur in the lesser curvature of the stomach; these ulcers require biopsy to rule out cancer after 6 weeks of conventional treatment.

Ascending colon: The ascending colon is located on the right side of the abdomen; fat-filled tags, or appendices epiploicae, are found on its surface. The transverse colon and part of the ascending colon are classified as intraperitoneal organs; sacculations, or haustra, are scattered along them and are visible on radiographs. The blood supply of both the ascending colon and the small intestine originates from the superior mesenteric artery. The cecum is the first part of the ascending colon; it is located at the connection between the colon and ileum of the small intestine. CT shows that the cecum connects to the vermiform appendix at its posterior and medial aspects with open communication between the cecum and the appendix. Any obstruction can cause appendicitis. Blood flow to the ascending colon originates from the ileocolic and right colic branches of the superior mesenteric artery; the blood supply from the cecum originates from the ileocecal branch of the superior mesenteric artery.

Descending colon: The descending colon is retroperitoneal, functioning to store stool and absorb water from stool. In combination of part of the transverse and sigmoid colon, it forms the embryological hindgut. CT shows that the descending colon is on the left side of the abdomen along the left paracolic gutter and is connected to the posterior abdominal wall from the splenic flexure to the pelvis. The blood supply to the descending colon originates from the left colic branch of the inferior mesenteric artery; the blood supply to the hindgut originates from the inferior mesenteric artery.

Transverse colon: The transverse colon is intraperitoneal, located by the transverse mesocolon, beginning at the hepatic flexure and ending at the splenic flexure. CT shows that the transverse colon is the longest part of the colon, dipping down to the pelvis, with a blood supply that originates at the middle colic artery, which is a branch of the superior mesenteric artery.

Duodenum second part: The first and shortest part of the small intestine, the duodenum second part is divided into 4 parts. CT shows that the first part is in the hepatoduodenal ligament; the second part is behind the transverse colon, anterior to the right kidney, and inferior to the liver. The blood supply originates from the superior pancreaticoduodenal artery, a branch of the celiac artery, and the inferior pancreaticoduodenal artery, a branch of the superior mesenteric artery.

Duodenum third part: The duodenum third part is about 2 inches long. It is the transverse part of the duodenum and is connected to the fourth and last part of the duodenum. It is held in place by the ligament of Treitz, which connects the duodenum to the right crus of the diaphragm.

Small intestine: As the longest part of the gastrointestinal tract, the small intestine forms the embryological midgut and is divided into the duodenum, jejunum, and ileum. CT shows the small intestine in the center of the abdomen with the colon at the superior and lateral edge. Multiple dilated loops of small intestine with air-fluid levels appear when the small bowel is obstructed by adhesions or hernias when the patient sits upright. The blood supply of the small intestine originates in the superior mesenteric artery. Cross-sectional images taken after the administration of a barium contrast agent show valvulae circulares of mucosa and white coloration caused by the filling of the small intestine with a barium contrast agent. The small intestine aids in digestion and absorption of protein and carbohydrates, and the terminal ileum allows the small intestine to absorb vitamin B12, bile salts, and fatty acids.

Cecum: As the first part of the large intestine, the cecum is approximately 7 cm long and receives its blood supply from the ileocolic artery, a branch of the superior mesenteric artery. CT shows that the cecum is in the right lower quadrant below the ascending colon; a part of it is attached to the appendix. The ileocecal valve of the cecum is unique because it is usually incompetent and allows the introduction of contrast material into the ileum (the last part of the small intestine) through the lower gastrointestinal tract. Usually encased by peritoneum, the cecum is mobile and can be a site of volvulus when chronic constipation causes movement of the cecum toward the left upper quadrant. Typical CT shows the cecum as a bird's peak sign, although an enlarged cecum can have a diameter of more than 10 cm.

Appendix: Attached to the cecum approximately 2.5 cm below the ileocecal junction, the appendix is about 8 cm long and can be longer and narrower in children than in adults. The appendix is thought to be a vestigial organ; it has no known function. The appendix is surrounded by mesentery of terminal ileum, or mesoappendix, which is where the blood supply for the appendix originates. CT shows that the appendix is located behind the cecum or behind the ascending colon; the base of the organ is two-thirds of the way from the umbilicus to the anterior superior iliac spine, or McBurney's point. Appendicitis is an inflammation of the appendix considered to be caused by obstruction with feces; it is more common in children than in adults.

<u>Vascular</u>

Inferior mesenteric artery: As the third branch of the abdominal aorta, the inferior mesenteric artery provides blood supply to the embryological hindgut organs: the distal transverse colon, the sigmoid colon, and the descending colon. The inferior mesenteric artery branches into the superior rectal, left colic, rectosigmoid, and sigmoid arteries; the ascending branches of the left colic artery form anastomoses to the middle colic artery as a branch of the superior mesenteric artery and form the marginal artery of Drummond.

Renal veins: The left and right renal veins originate from the aorta to travel to the superior mesenteric artery and join the IVC. The right renal vein is shorter than the left and travels anterior to the right renal artery. The left gonadal vein drains into the left renal vein; the right gonadal vein drains into the IVC.

Renal arteries: The right and left renal arteries originate from the abdominal aorta below the origin of the superior mesenteric artery. The right renal artery travels posterior to the IVC.

Splenic artery: The splenic artery is the largest branch of the celiac trunk because of the large volume of blood flow to the spleen. CT shows that the splenic artery travels posterior to the fundus of the stomach, providing a branch of the left gastro-omental artery to supply blood to the greater curvature of the stomach, and enters the hilum of the spleen, where it divides into 5 or more branches in the splenorenal ligament. Aneurysms may form in the gastro-omental artery; these aneurysms are identified by eggshell calcifications.

Celiac trunk: The celiac trunk has 3 main branches: the hepatic artery, the splenic artery, and the left gastric artery. CT shows that the celiac trunk originates from the anterior aspect of the aorta soon after entering the abdomen.

Common hepatic artery: The common hepatic artery supplies blood to several organs in the abdomen. CT shows that the gastroduodenal branch of the hepatic artery supplies the duodenum and wraps around the greater curvature of the stomach to supply the stomach; it also forms anastomoses to the gastro-omental artery, a branch of the splenic artery. Blood is also supplied to the liver through the proper hepatic artery, which branches off to the right gastric artery to supply blood to the lesser curvature of the stomach before forming an anastomosis with the left gastric artery.

Splenic vein: The splenic vein is formed by various veins draining the spleen at the hilum. CT shows that the splenic vein travels posterior to the body and tail of the pancreas before joining the inferior mesenteric vein and merging with the superior mesenteric vein to form the portal vein.

Common iliac arteries: The retroperitoneal common iliac arteries continue the abdominal aorta after it bifurcates in the abdomen. CT shows that the right and left common iliac arteries give rise to the internal and external iliac arteries in the pelvis. The right common iliac artery is located anterior to the right common iliac vein, and the common iliacs are crossed by the ureters anteriorly.

The common iliac veins form the IVC. Both veins are formed by internal and external iliac veins and drain the blood from the pelvis and the lower extremity. CT shows the common iliac veins posterior and to the right of the common iliac arteries. The iliac wing has a fossa that forms a portion of the posterior abdominal wall. CT shows that the ilium forms the top two-thirds of the hipbone and two-fifths of the acetabulum, the location of the head of the femur. The fossa of the iliac wing is an attachment point for many pelvic muscles.

External iliac vessels: The external iliac vessels are one of 2 bifurcations of the common iliac artery before it descends into the pelvis. CT shows that the external iliac artery provides the main blood supply to the lower limb and gives rise to the inferior epigastric and deep circumflex iliac arteries before becoming the femoral artery.

CT of the Pelvis

Urinary bladder

The urinary bladder is a hollow muscle that functions to hold urine. CT shows that the adult urinary bladder is located posterior and superior to the pubic bones in the pelvis and extends to the abdomen when full. In infants, the urinary bladder is located in the abdomen. The bladder is distensible with folds, or rugae, except in the triangular-shaped area at the base of the bladder, the trigone, at which location the bladder is smooth.

Colorectal

Sigmoid colon: The sigmoid colon is the portion of the colon that is encased in mesentery called sigmoid mesocolon. It is located between the descending colon and the rectum. CT shows that the sigmoid colon is located in the upper part of the pelvis, inferior to the small intestines. It serves to store stool before defecation and is a common site for colon cancer.

Rectum: The rectum is the final section of the colon, considered to be retroperitoneal because it is only partially covered with peritoneum and is continuous with the anal canal. CT shows that the rectum is located between the sigmoid colon and the anus, posterior to the urinary bladder in males and posterior to the vagina and the uterus in females. The middle rectal branches of the inferior iliac vessels and the inferior mesenteric artery supply blood to the rectum.

Reproductive organs

Seminal vesicle: The seminal vesicle is found only in males; it serves to secrete a thick alkaline fluid mixed with sperm as the fluid passes into ejaculatory ducts and is secreted during orgasm. CT shows that the seminal vesicle is located posterior to the urinary bladder. The seminal vesicle duct joins the ductus deferens to form the ejaculatory duct, which joins the prostatic urethra at the posterior end.

Prostate gland: The prostate gland produces a milky fluid that composes approximately 20% of the ejaculate. CT shows that the prostate is walnut-sized and is located beneath the urinary bladder. It has lateral and middle lobes. The prostate gland is a common site for cancer in men older than 75. Prostate cancer is a slow-growing cancer that causes enlargement of the lateral lobe, which may be palpated during rectal examination.

Base of the penis: The base of the penis comprises the root bulb and the bulbospongiosus muscle. CT shows that the bulb is penetrated by the urethra.

Vagina: The vagina creates a thick fluid for lubrication during sexual activity and serves as a canal leading from the external orifice of the genital canal to the uterus.

Uterus: The uterus is a muscular organ that serves to contain and nourish the young during physical and neurological development before birth.

Ovaries: The ovaries occur in pairs in most females and act to create and store eggs that are to be fertilized during sexual intercourse. The ovaries also produce hormones that are related to proper growth and development in young girls and to proper maintenance of the hormone cycle in adult women who experience menstruation. CT shows that the uterus is easily visualized in females of all ages. It is superior to the urinary bladder, although the ovaries are less easily visualized in younger females.

Musculoskeletal CT

CT scanning has been used extensively in musculoskeletal imaging and radiology since the development and accessibility of multidetector scanners; musculoskeletal imaging has also been improved by the ability of the system to scan the patient's body in very thin slice collimations with multiplanar reformations. The spine and other osseous body parts and structures, including the extremities and the pelvis, can be easily evaluated with CT. Such evaluations allow for treatment based on high-quality diagnostic images of the thoracic, cervical, and lumbar spines in the axial plane when combined with sagittal coronal reformations. More sensitive than plain film radiography, CT is the preferred method of evaluating trauma patients with musculoskeletal injuries and is quickly becoming the diagnostic standard in many trauma facilities.

Lower extremity

Psoas muscle: The psoas muscle extends from the transverse processes of the lumbar vertebrae to the lesser trochanter of the femur; it is involved in flexing the thigh at the hip. CT shows that the psoas muscle is in a retroperitoneal position, although it is considered a muscle of the posterior abdominal wall. The psoas muscle has major and minor counterparts and is important in the development and health of other abdominal muscles and the pancreas.

Gluteus maximus muscle: The gluteus maximus muscle acts to extend the thigh and assists in the lateral rotation of the thigh. CT shows that the gluteus maximus muscle originates from the external surface of the ala of the ilium and the dorsum of the sacrum. It attaches to the iliotibial tract and the lateral condyle of the tibia. The gluteus maximus muscle also raises the trunk from a flexed position and is used in jumping, climbing, running, and walking. Its main enervation comes from the inferior gluteal nerve.

Gluteus medius muscle: The gluteus medius muscle is deep to the gluteus maximus muscle and is used in abducting the hip joint and maintaining the tilt of the pelvis during walking. CT shows that the muscle originates from the external surface of the ilium and attaches to the lateral surface of the greater trochanter of the femur. Its enervation comes from the superior gluteal nerve.

Gluteus minimus muscle: The gluteus minimus muscle is the smallest and most deeply located gluteus muscle. Its functions are similar to those of the medius, although it plays a larger role in the rotation of thigh muscles medially. CT shows that the gluteus minimus muscle is attached to the external surface of the ilium and to the anterior aspect of the greater trochanter of the femur, with enervation from the superior gluteal nerve.

Piriformis muscle: The piriformis muscle functions to laterally rotate and abduct the thigh. CT shows that the piriformis muscle is located in the posterior pelvis and originates from the second through fourth sacral segments before inserting on the greater trochanter of the femur. A pear-shaped muscle, the piriformis muscle plays a role similar to that of the obturator internus in moving the femur.

Femoral head: The femoral head forms the part of the femur that fits into the acetabulum of the pelvis. CT shows that the femoral head has a center, or fovea, at which the ligament is attached to the head of the femur and the body through the femoral neck.

Greater trochanter: The greater trochanter is a large projection of the femur that is located at the union of the neck and the body of the femur. CT shows that the greater trochanter serves as an important attachment junction for large muscles, including the gluteus medius and the gluteus minimus.

Rectus femoris muscle: The rectus femoris muscle works with 3 other muscles to make up the quadriceps muscles, one of the largest muscle groups in the body. CT shows that the rectus femoris muscle originates from the anterior inferior iliac spine to travel down the thigh and attach to the top of the patella. Enervated by the femoral nerve, the rectus femoris muscle contributes to the extension of the knee joint in such activities as jumping, climbing, and rising from a chair.

Gracilis muscle: The gracilis muscle is the weakest of the adductor muscle group in the thigh and functions to adduct the thigh and flex the leg. CT shows that the gracilis muscle is in a medial position in the thigh and knees while the knee joint is crossed. It receives its enervation through the obturator nerve.

Sartorius muscle: The sartorius muscle is strap-like and functions to flex, abduct, and laterally rotate the thigh at the hip joint. CT shows that the sartorius muscle originates from the anterior superior iliac spine before inserting into the superior part of the medial surface of the tibia. It is a superficial muscle of the anterior thigh and receives enervation from the branches of the femoral nerve.

Adductor magnus muscle: The adductor magnus muscle is the largest muscle of the adductor group in the thigh. CT shows that the adductor magnus muscle originates from the inferior ramus of the pubic bones and attaches to the gluteal tuberosity and the adductor tubercle of the femur. With 2 heads, the adductor magnus muscle functions to adduct and flex the thigh as an adductor and hamstring part. It is enervated by the obturator and sciatic nerves.

Adductor longus muscle: The adductor longus muscle functions with the adductor magnus to adduct the thigh and is enervated by the obturator nerve. CT shows that the adductor longus muscle is the most anterior muscle in the adductor group in the thigh. It originates from the body of the pubis and attaches to the pectineal line and the proximal part of the linea aspera of the femur.

Vastus lateralis muscle: The vastus lateralis muscle is one of 4 muscles in the quadriceps group; it functions to extend the lower leg at the knee joint. CT shows that the vastus lateralis muscle is on the lateral side of the thigh and originates from the greater trochanter of the femur before attaching to the patellar ligament.

Vastus intermedius muscle: The vastus intermedius muscle is another of the quadriceps group. CT shows that the vastus intermedius muscle originates from the anterior and lateral surface of the femur and attaches to the patellar ligament.

Vastus medialis muscle: The vastus medialis muscle functions to extend the lower leg at the knee joint and is the most medial muscle in the quadriceps group. CT shows that the vastus medialis muscle originates from the intertrochanteric line of the femur and attaches to the patellar ligament.

Semimembranosus and semitendinosus muscles: The semimembranosus and semitendinosus muscles, along with the biceps femoris, comprise the hamstring muscles and work together to extend the thigh and flex the leg, as well as medially rotate the tibia. CT shows that the semimembranosus and semitendinosus muscles are located in the posterior aspect of the thigh, where they cross the knee and insert the tibia. Strenuous exercise, including running or kicking, can tear the fibers of the hamstring muscles; such tears lead to the development of hematomas and intense muscular pain.

Tensor fascia latae: The tensor fascia latae is a short, strap-like muscle with fibers that pass downward and backward before inserting on the iliotibial tract just below the level of the greater trochanter. CT shows that the tensor fascia latae arises from the anterior part of the iliac crest near the anterior superior iliac spine but lies just anterior to the anterior border of the gluteus medius.

Pectineus muscle: The pectineus muscle forms a significant part of the femoral triangle. CT shows that the pectineus muscle is just medial to the iliopsoas. It arises from the pecten of the pubis with the bone anterior to the pecten, and it inserting on the posterior aspect of the femur on the pectineal line. Arising from the femoral artery or the profunda femoris, the medial femoral circumflex artery passes back between the pectineus muscle and the iliopsoas, and the femoral vessels are located just in front of the pectineus muscles.

Spine

CT is successful for scanning the spine and vertebrae and can detect tumors, deformities, a narrowing of the spinal canal as seen with spinal stenosis, or any other problems that might exist in the spine. CT of the spine has been instrumental in assisting practitioners in diagnosing treatable diseases or growths and in determining possible treatments for other conditions. Spinal CT scans are used to detect a herniated disc in the spine and to detect osteoporosis and determine the complications associated with it. CT can also be used to guide a needle during tissue biopsy or drainage of an abscess.

Disadvantages of CT for spinal cord imaging: In emergency situations, CT can verify the presence of trauma after injury to the head or upper torso, aiding practitioners in their initial review and response to damage. However, the success of CT is limited in evaluating the stability of the spinal cord because the images of the spinal cord obtained by CT are satisfactory at best but do not provide comparably effective images of the central canal contents. Thus, the spinal cord cannot be well visualized. Some practitioners have achieved success by using lumbar puncture to administer intrathecal contract agents that can facilitate visualization during CT scanning, but this type of procedure has mostly been replaced by MRI because it is more sensitive and less invasive in imaging the spinal cord.

Vertebral body: The vertebral body is the large anterior part of each vertebra; the vertebral bodies are larger in the lower regions of the lumbar area to bear the weight of the upper body. CT shows that the vertebral bodies are separated by the intervertebral discs, cushions of fibrous tissue composed of the annulus fibrosis and nucleus pulposus.

Erector spinae muscle: The erector spinae muscle is located on each side of the spinal column. It serves to extend the vertebral column with its 3 muscles, all of which originate from a tendon located in the posterior portion of the iliac crest. CT scan shows that the erector spinae muscle is attached to the transverse processes of the cervical vertebrae and the mastoid process.

Rectus abdominis muscle: The rectus abdominis muscle is the principal muscle of the anterior abdominal wall. CT shows that it runs vertically from the xiphoid process to the pubic symphysis and the pubic crest, where it divides into 2 components in the center of the abdomen by the linea alba. The rectus abdominis muscle is wide in the superior location and narrow on its course to the pubic symphysis. It is enclosed by a rectus sheath to compress the abdomen during coughing and defecating and to stabilize the pelvis during walking.

External oblique muscle: The external oblique muscle originates from the external surfaces of the fifth through twelfth ribs to attach to the linea alba, the pubic tubercle, and the anterior half of the iliac crest. This muscle is the most superficial of the 3 flat anterior abdominal wall muscles. The external oblique muscle compresses the abdomen during defecation and parturition.

Internal oblique muscle: The internal oblique muscle originates from the anterior two-thirds of the iliac crest before inserting into the inferior borders of the twelfth ribs and the linea alba. CT shows that the internal oblique muscle lies in the middle of the anterior abdominal wall muscles with an origin at the lateral half of the inguinal ligament. The internal oblique muscle compresses the abdomen during defecation and parturition and also supports the organs of the abdomen.

Transversus abdominis muscle: The transversus abdominis muscle medially contributes to the formation of the rectus sheath, which encases the rectus abdominis muscle. A CT scan shows that the transversus abdominis muscle originates from the internal surfaces of the seventh through twelfth costal cartilages and the iliac crest. It acts as the lateral third of the inguinal ligament before attaching with the internal and external obliques to form the linea alba. The transversus abdominis muscle is the deepest anterior abdominal wall muscle.

Quadratus lumborum muscle: The quadratus lumborum muscle extends and flexes the vertebral column. CT shows that the quadratus lumborum muscle is being lateral and posterior to the psoas muscles and adjacent to the transverse processes of the lumbar vertebrae. It originates from the medial half of the inferior border of the twelfth rib before inserting into the iliolumbar ligament and the internal lip of the iliac crest.

Pelvic girdle

Sacrum: The sacrum supports the pelvis and transmits the weight of the body into the legs through the sacroiliac joints. Formed by 5 sacral vertebral fused together, the sacrum is one of 3 bones that form the pelvis. The sacrum has 4 pairs of foramina on each side, which providing exit points for the dorsal and ventral sacral nerves. The 5 sacral vertebrae do not begin to fuse until the patient reaches the age of 20.

Inferior pubic ramus: The inferior pubic ramus is part of the pubic bone. CT shows that the inferior pubic ramus passes posteriorly and inferiorly to connect with the ramus of the ischium to complete the formation of half of the pubic arch.

Iliacus muscle: The iliacus muscle originates from the iliac crest, the iliac fossa, and the ala of the sacrum. It is involved in the process of flexing the thigh at the hip joint. CT shows that the iliacus muscle is being located lateral to the psoas major muscle and is attached to the body of the femur as it exists below the trochanter.

Ischial spine: The ischial spine projects medially as part of the ischium and separate the greater sciatic notch superiorly from the lesser sciatic notch. CT shows that the ischial spine is above the greater sciatic notch and the ischial tuberosity.

Ischiorectal fossa: The ischiorectal fossa houses the internal pudendal artery and nerve. It also contains soft fat pads, or ischioanal pads, and acts as a site of infection that originates from the anal sinuses or rectal abscess. CT shows that the ischiorectal fossa has with walls that are bound laterally by the ischium, medially by the anal canal, posteriorly by the sacrotuberous ligament and the gluteus maximus, and anteriorly by the urogenital diaphragm.

Symphysis pubis: The symphysis pubis is a tough cartilage joining the bodies of the 2 pubic bones. It is thicker in women than in men so that more mobility may be realized in the pelvic bones, allowing a greater diameter of the pelvic cavity during parturition. CT shows that the symphysis pubis has an articular surface covered by a thin layer of hyaline cartilage.

Ischial tuberosity: The ischial tuberosity is the most inferior portion of the ischium and bears the weight of a body when it is sitting on a chair. CT shows that the ischial tuberosity is normally covered by the gluteus maximus when the thigh is extended and is uncovered by the gluteus maximus when the thigh is flexed.

Internal obturator muscle: The internal obturator muscle originates from the ilium and the ischium and is enervated by the obturator internus nerve. It works with the piriformis muscle to rotate the thigh and to hold the head of the femur in place at the acetabulum. It forms most of the lateral wall of the pelvis, traversing through the lesser sciatic foramen, and attaches to the greater trochanter of the femur.

External obturator muscle: The external obturator muscle originates from the obturator foramen in the superior medial portion of the thigh and is enervated by the obturator internus nerve. It crosses posteriorly to the femur before attaching at the trochanteric fossa. Like the internal obturator muscle, the external obturator muscle rotates the thigh and holds the head of the femur in the acetabulum.

Vascular

Common femoral artery: The common femoral artery continues the external iliac vessels below the inguinal ligament. CT shows that the common femoral artery is lateral to the femoral vein and medial to the femoral nerve, best represented by NAVL, a mnemonic for the location of the structures in the femoral triangle from most to least lateral: nerve, artery, vein, lymphatics. This artery is a good site for arterial blood gas (ABG) measurements, whereas the vein can be used for central line placement. The artery is lateral to the vein, and the artery's pulse is usually palpable.

Superficial femoral artery: The superficial femoral artery (SFA) provides blood supply to the lower legs and is formed by the bifurcation of the common femoral artery. The superficial femoral artery runs deep to the sartorius muscle before continuing to the adductor canal formed by the adductor magnus muscle. CT shows that the SFA leaves the canal at the adductor hiatus, or Hunter's canal, and enters the popliteal fossa to continue as the popliteal artery to supply blood to the lower leg. This positioning of the artery makes the SFA most susceptible to gunshot wounds and lacerations; it is also a common site of atherosclerotic plaque formation in patients with atherosclerotic artery disease. A blocked SFA causes leg pains that are relieved only by rest. Balloon angioplasty can be used to open the clogged vessel.

Focus of Questions

Sectional anatomy

Sagittal plane

The sagittal plane is the imaginary plane that complements the long axis used to divide the body into right and left sections. The sagittal plane is used by practitioners and researchers during study and analysis.

Coronal plane

The coronal plane is the imaginary plane that divides the body into front and back, or anterior and posterior, sections. The coronal plane is used by practitioners and researchers during study and analysis.

Axial plane

Axial refers to any body part or measurement that is parallel to the dividing line, or long axis, of the body. The axial plane is the imaginary plane that differentiates between the sagittal and coronal planes, that is, between the right and left sections and between the front and back sections.

Landmarks

Superior sagittal sinus: The superior sagittal sinus (SSS) is located at the attached convex margin of the falx cerebri. CT shows that the SSS begins in a posterior direction at the foramen cecum with grooves on the inner surface of the frontal bone, adjacent parts of the parietal bones, and the inner aspect of the occipital bones. In cross-section it appears triangular, and it gradually enlarges in its posterior progression.

Falx cerebri: The falx cerebri is a strong arched membrane with a sickle-like shape. CT shows that the falx cerebri extends downward vertically in the longitudinal fissure between the cerebral hemispheres.

Frontal lobe: The frontal lobe crosses from the frontal pole to the central sulcus. CT shows that the frontal lobe lies mostly in the anterior cranial fossa; its lower surface is shallowly concave to correspond to the orbital roof. The lateral sulcus separates the frontal lobe from the temporal lobe.

Parietal lobe: The parietal lobe is confluent with the temporal and occipital lobes at the end of the sulcus on the lateral surface of the hemisphere. CT shows that the parietal lobe is located between the frontal, occipital, and temporal lobes and is separated from the frontal lobe by the central sulcus.

Central sulcus: The central sulcus forms the boundary between the frontal and parietal lobes and separates the primary sensory cortex at the posterior from the primary motor cortex at the anterior.

Superior frontal sulcus: The superior frontal sulcus exists as a continuous sulcus to separate the superior frontal gyrus from the middle frontal gyrus.

Precentral gyrus: The precentral gyrus serves as the primary motor region of the cerebral cortex and is bounded by the precentral sulcus and the central sulcus.

Postcentral gyrus: The postcentral gyrus runs parallel to the precentral gyrus and serves as the primary somesthetic cortex so that general sensory projections can be represented in a somatotropic pattern.

Cingulated gyrus: An arched convolution, the cingulated gyrus lies entirely adjacent to the corpus callosum, from which it is separated by the sulcus of the corpus callosum.

Middle frontal gyrus: The middle frontal gyrus is a wide convolution extending anteroinferiorly from the precentral gyrus. It is bounded by the superior frontal sulcus above and the inferior frontal sulcus below.

Superior frontal gyrus: The superior frontal gyrus is a wide, uneven convolution extending to the medial surface of the hemisphere and lying above the superior frontal sulcus.

Midbrain: The midbrain is the portion of the neurotaxis that occurs between the pons and thalamus. Also known as the mesencephalon, the midbrain is a short, constricted segment of the brainstem shown on CT as measuring only 2 cm in length.

Mamillary bodies: The mamillary bodies create prominent projections on each side of the ventral surface of the posterior hypothalamus as it is located near the midline.

Temporal lobe: The temporal lobe lies below the lateral sulcus; its back end is continuous with the occipital lobe.

Cerebral aqueduct: The cerebral aqueduct connects the third and fourth ventricle with no choroids plexus. Any blockage results in hydrocephalus.

Cerebral peduncle: The cerebral peduncle forms half of the midbrain and can be used interchangeably.

Optic tract: The optic tract winds obliquely from the chiasma to the cerebral peduncle across the undersurface. Medial fibers in the optic nerve cross in the chiasma and continue on the other side, whereas the lateral fibers remain uncrossed and continue to the brain on the same side.

Trapezius muscle: The trapezius muscle is a large superficial back muscle that attaches the pectoral girdle to the vertebral column and the skull. CT shows that this muscle can elevate, depress, rotate, and retract the scapula.

Left and right clavicles: The left and right clavicles extend horizontally at the base of the neck from the acromion of the scapula to the manubrium of the sternum, with medial ends articulating with the sternum at the sternoclavicular joint. CT shows that the clavicles attach the upper limbs to the skeleton and provide a basis for major muscle groups.

Subscapularis muscle: The subscapularis muscle is one of 4 muscles in the rotator cuff that provide stability for the shoulder joint by holding the top of the humerus in the glenoid cavity of the scapula. CT shows that the subscapularis muscle is anterior to the scapula and posterior to the serratus anterior muscle; it inserts in the lesser tubercle of the humerus.

Infraspinatus muscle: The infraspinatus muscle is the second muscle in the rotator cuff, originating from the dorsal aspect of the scapula to insert into the greater tubercle of the humerus. CT shows that it is inferior to the spine of the scapula; it rotates the arm and stabilizes the shoulder joint.

Supraspinatus muscle: The supraspinatus muscle is the third muscle in the rotator cuff, originating in the supraspinatus fossa of the scapula, which is above the spine of the scapula. CT shows that the infraspinatus muscle inserts into the superior aspect of the great tubercle of the humerus, thereby helping to stabilize the shoulder joint.

Teres minor muscle: The teres minor muscle is the fourth muscle in the rotator cuff, originating from the superior part of the lateral border of the scapula and inserting into the greater tubercle of the humerus. CT shows that the teres minor is below the spine of the scapula and sits superior to the teres major muscle.

Pectoralis major muscle: The pectoralis major muscle sits in the anterior thorax, enclosed by a fascial sheath forming the axillary fascia. CT shows that the pectoralis major is superficial to the pectoralis minor and serratus anterior muscles, although the pectoralis major inserts into the greater tubercle of the humerus.

Pectoralis minor muscle: The pectoralis minor muscle is located deeper than the pectoralis major and originates from the costal cartilage of ribs 3 through 5 to insert on the coracoid process of the scapula. CT shows that the pectoralis minor pulls the scapula inferiorly and anteriorly to stabilize it.

Serratus anterior muscle: The serratus anterior muscle is located in the lateral aspect of the thorax and originates from the external surface of the lateral parts of ribs 1 through 8, inserting on the anterior surface of the medial border of the scapula. CT shows that the serratus anterior sits anterior to the subscapularis muscle and pulls the scapula toward the thorax in a forward swing.

Latissimus dorsi muscle: The latissimus dorsi muscle is a large back muscle that extends from the lower back to the crest of the lesser tubercle and the intertubercular groove of the humerus. It originates from the spinous process of the inferior 6 thoracic vertebrae and the last 4 ribs. CT shows that the latissimus dorsi lies inferior to the teres major and minor muscles and is used to extend, abduct, and medially rotate the humerus.

Erector spinae muscles: The erector spinae muscles sit in a group of 3 parallel to the vertebral column laterally on both sides of the spinous process of each vertebral process. CT shows that the erector spinae muscles extend from the cervical vertebrae down to the tubercles of ribs 9 and 10.

Left subclavian artery: The left subclavian artery is the third branch of the ascending aorta and rises to enter the root of the neck toward the upper limbs. CT shows that it divides the subclavian artery into 3 parts.

Distal and right subclavian arteries: The distal and right subclavian arteries form the axillary artery once it passes the first rib, at which point the axillary artery becomes the brachia artery. CT shows that the distal and right subclavian arteries cross the inferior border of the teres major muscles.

Left common carotid artery: The left common carotid artery is encased in the carotid sheath and originates from the arch of the aorta to ascend in the neck before dividing into the external and internal carotid at the superior border of the thyroid cartilage. CT shows that the left common carotid artery is lateral to the internal jugular veins.

Right common carotid artery: The right common carotid artery arises from the brachiocephalic trunks as a branch paired with the subclavian artery. CT shows that the right common carotid artery is located at the bifurcation of the internal and external carotid vessels.

Internal jugular veins: The internal jugular veins drain the blood supply of the brain and face as the largest veins in the neck, starting at the jugular foramen and traveling through the neck. CT shows that the jugular veins are superficial, medial to the sternocleidomastoid muscle, deep to the medial end of the clavicle, lateral to the common carotid artery, and anterior to the vagus nerve. The right internal jugular vein is usually larger than the left because of the larger volume of blood entering the vein from the sigmoid sinus.

Scapula: The scapula and the clavicles make up the pectoral girdle and connect the upper limbs to the axial skeleton. CT shows that the scapula sits in the posterior aspect of the thorax, with the spine on the posterior surface forming the acromion, which wraps around the scapula superiorly to articulate with the lateral end of the clavicles at the acromial-clavicular joint.

First rib: The first rib is the most curved and widest rib, providing an attachment point for the anterior scalene muscle and connecting the upper limb to the subclavian artery and vein and the brachial plexus. CT shows that the first rib is anterior to the subclavian vein, which travels anterior to the anterior scalene muscle. All of these structures are posterior to the clavicle.

Second rib: The second rib is longer than the first, and CT shows that the second rib is not as curved as the first rib.

Manubrium of the sternum: The manubrium of the sternum articulates both the clavicle and the first rib as the broadly shaped superior portion of the sternum. CT shows that the superior aspect of the manubrium has a notch that makes it easily palpable.

Body of the sternum: The body of the sternum articulates with ribs 2 through 7 to form the anterior and medial parts of the thorax. CT shows that the body of the sternum is inferior to, longer than, and narrower than the manubrium.

Xiphoid process of the sternum: The xiphoid process of the sternum is the most inferior part of the sternum because it is the short and pointed end. CT shows that middle-aged patients no longer have a cartilaginous xiphoid process because it has begun to ossify and join with the body of the sternum.

Aortic arch: The aortic arch is located at the level of the sternal angle as a continuation of the ascending aorta, found in the middle mediastinum. CT shows that the aorta arches over the root of the left lung to travel posteriorly and to the left of the trachea and esophagus. It then becomes the descending aorta and travels in the posterior mediastinum.

Ascending aorta: The ascending aorta is the first part of the aorta with its first branch as the brachiocephalic trunk. CT shows that the ascending aorta begins in the anterior mediastinum and arches back toward the posterior mediastinum. It lies to the left of the superior vena cava and to the right of the pulmonary trunk.

Descending aorta: The descending aorta continues the arch of the aorta, piercing the diaphragm to enter the abdomen. CT shows that it lies to the left of the vertebral column, posterior to the esophagus, to the left of the thoracic duct, and anterior to the hemiazygous vein.

Azygous vein: The azygous vein drains blood from the posterior thorax and abdomen; it originates posteriorly to the inferior vena cava and renal vein. CT shows that the azygous vein is posterior to the thoracic duct and to the right of the vertebral column, with the hemiazygous system of veins to the left.

Arch of the azygous: The arch of the azygous is located over the root of the right lung, and CT shows that it empties into the superior vena cava.

Right brachiocephalic vein: The right brachiocephalic vein is formed by the right internal jugular vein and the right subclavian vein behind the medial end of the right clavicle. CT shows that the right brachiocephalic vein is only half the length of the left brachiocephalic vein.

Left brachiocephalic vein: The left brachiocephalic vein travels to the right to connect with the right brachiocephalic vein behind the manubrium of the sternum. CT shows that the left brachiocephalic vein is posterior to the thymus and the receiving end of the thoracic duct, which drains lymph from the pelvis and the lower extremities to empty into the left brachiocephalic vein.

Superior vena cava: The superior vena cava is formed by the union of the right and left brachiocephalic veins. CT shows that the superior vena cava is a tributary draining blood from the head and upper extremities.

Thymus gland: The thymus gland is more visible in children than in adults and plays an active role in the development of lymphocytes in the immune system. CT shows that the thymus gland is located at the anterior portion of the superior mediastinum and is the site of origin for the carcinoma malignant thymoma, which is part of the disease myasthenia gravis.

Teres major muscle: The teres major muscle is not part of the rotator cuff series but works to stabilize the shoulder joint by holding the head of the humerus in the glenoid cavity. CT shows that the teres major muscle sits inferior to the teres minor muscle, originating from the inferior angle of the scapula and inserting into the intertubercular groove of the humerus.

Left subclavian vein: The left subclavian vein or axillary vein originates from the brachial vein to drain the blood supply from the upper limbs. It travels over the first rib to connect with the internal jugular vein to form the brachiocephalic vein. CT shows that the left subclavian or axillary vein is posterior to the clavicle but anterior to the anterior scalene.

Brachiocephalic artery: The brachiocephalic artery is the largest branch of the aorta. CT shows that the brachiocephalic artery connects with the right subclavian and right common carotid vessels at a point posterior to the right sternoclavicular joint.

Inferior vena cava: The inferior vena cava is one of 3 veins draining into the right atrium, acting as a tributary to the iliac, mesenteric, pelvic, hepatic, and left renal veins. CT shows that it is to the right of the abdominal aorta and ascends to the abdomen at a posterior-to-anterior position to the aorta before piercing the diaphragm. The IVC traverses its own foramen, located at T-8, in the diaphragm to enter the thorax.

Pulmonary trunk: The pulmonary trunk is the outlet of the right ventricle that carries deoxygenated blood to the lungs. CT shows that the pulmonary trunk is approximately 5 cm long and is the origin of the right and left pulmonary arteries.

Right pulmonary artery: The right pulmonary artery returns deoxygenated blood from the body and connects to the ascending aorta and superior vena cava. CT shows that it is inferior to the arch of the aorta, posterior to the superior vena cava, and posterior to the pulmonary vein in the right hilum.

Left pulmonary artery: The left pulmonary artery provides an avenue for blood to go toward the body without entering the high-resistance circulation of the lungs. CT shows that it is connected to the arch of the aorta and that the left recurrent laryngeal nerve loops around the arch of the aorta to return to the neck.

Thoracic duct: The thoracic duct drains lymph from the pelvis, the abdomen, the left side of the thorax, and the lower extremities. It originates from the cisterna chili to eventually drain into the left brachiocephalic vein. CT shows that the thoracic duct is anterior to the vertebral column and curves to the left before reaching the thorax.

Carina of the trachea: The carina of the trachea is the area at which the trachea bifurcates into right and left mainstem bronchi to continue its travel vertically at the carina. CT scans show that the carina of the trachea is located at the arch of the aorta, although any distortion of the normal appearance could indicate enlarged lymph nodes or other pathology at the carina.

Abdominal aorta: The abdominal aorta is retroperitoneal and bifurcates into common iliac vessels near the level of the umbilicus. CT shows that the abdominal aorta is anterior to the vertebrae; it traverses through the diaphragm at the foramen at T-12 and stays to the left of the IVC. Aneurysms that form in the abdominal aorta below the origin of the renal vessels in elderly patients cause back pain and a pulsatile abdominal mass.

Portal vein: The portal vein is formed at the union of the inferior mesenteric, superior mesenteric, and splenic veins; it is sheathed in the hepatoduodenal ligament with the common hepatic artery and the common bile duct to form the portal triad that enters the portal hepatis. CT shows that the portal vein is anterior to the IVC. It is a site for thrombosis in patients with an increased risk of clotting.

Superior mesenteric artery: The superior mesenteric artery is the second branch of the abdominal aorta; it provides blood to the duodenum, jejunum, and ileum. CT shows that the superior mesenteric artery travels between the head and uncinate process to the left of the superior mesenteric vein.

Superior mesenteric vein: The superior mesenteric vein (SMV) drains blood from the small intestine before emptying into the portal vein. CT shows that the SMV travels through the pancreas between the uncinate process and the head to the right of the superior mesenteric artery.

Pathology recognition:

Recognizing damage by reviewing radiologic features: Most practitioners are familiar with the use of CT and MRI to define abnormalities and can recommend corrections based on the results of such imaging. All practitioners should be able to identify the radiologic features of a normal adult or pediatric skull as evidenced on modern AP, lateral, and occipital projections. These features include the coronal, sagittal, sphenosquamosal, and lambdoidal sutures. Practitioners should also be able to recognize the innominate and mendosal sutures and the sphenooccipital synchondrosis associated with newborns and infants, as well as inner table vascular grooves, including the anterior and posterior divisions of the middle meningeal artery, the sphenoparietal venous groove, the transverse and sigmoid dural venous sinuses, and the intradiploic vascular channels and lakes. All of these features can be analyzed through scanning and tests and should be documented in the patient's records.

Recognizing fractures: Radiographic images can demonstrate skull fractures or other abnormal developments within the head. Various tests can show physiologic intracranial calcifications in the pineal gland, the habenular commissure, the falx, the choroids plexus of lateral ventricles, the dura, and the clinopetrosal ligament. Some practitioners will be able to recognize the distinctive radiographic characteristics associated with various types of skull fractures, vascular grooves, and intradiploic vascular channels and to identify the predictable anatomic locations of sutures, inner table arterial grooves, and other dural sinus channels. In this analysis, practitioners should avoid misreading the results because artifacts can be mistaken for pathologic abnormalities, especially on lateral skull radiographs.

Carotid artery stenosis: Also called carotid artery disease, carotid artery stenosis is the narrowing of the carotid arteries, which are the main arteries in the neck that supply blood to the brain. Carotid artery stenosis is a serious risk factor for an ischemic stroke, the most common form of stroke. The stenosis is usually initiated by a blood clot that blocks an artery. Plaque in the blood vessel causes the narrowing and is formed by a build-up of cholesterol, fat, and other substances in the inner lining of the artery; this process is called atherosclerosis. Carotid artery stenosis may occur with no presenting symptoms, although practitioners can hear an abnormal sound, or bruit, from the artery through a stethoscope. An ultrasound probe may also be placed on the side of the neck near the carotid arteries to detect the stenosis in a process called ultrasonography.

CT can provide a detailed view of the carotid arteries and is usually performed after other in-office tests have yielded positive results. In a process called carotid endarterectomy, practitioners can treat the carotid artery stenosis to remove the plaque that causes the carotid artery to narrow. The indications for carotid endarterectomy are based on the patient's overall condition and the degree of the stenosis. Patients whose arteries are narrowed, or stenosed, by 70 percent or more can usually benefit from carotid endarterectomy, whereas patients with a narrowing of less than 50 percent can usually benefit from medication, such as anticoagulant or antiplatelet agents, that can reduce the risk of ischemic stroke. Some practitioners recommend carotid angioplasty, which involves the use of balloons or stents to open the narrowed artery.

> **Review Video:** Anticoagulants, Thrombolytics, and Antiplatelets
> Visit mometrix.com/academy and enter code: 711284

Coronary calcification: An ECG tracing, allowing for a delay time of 80% of the recovery interval, can be used to analyze and define the diastolic phase of the heart. Multislice CT with a 500-ms rotation time provides practitioners with images that have a temporal resolution of 250-ms. Four adjacent slices with the perspective ECG trigger produce a typical scan of coronary arteries in about 15 seconds. The amount of calcium is scored on the basis of the Agatston scoring algorithm, developed for EBCT scoring, and the CT threshold score of 130 HU is selected with a coronary score for each main branch of the coronary artery (i.e., right, circumflex, left main, left anterior). The computer measures the calcification and multiplies measurement by a predetermined factor based on the peak attenuation value of the particular lesion. This multiplication yields a score that falls into one of 4 categories: no calcification, minimal calcification, moderate calcification, or extensive calcification. Higher scores suggest myocardial events.

Epidural hematoma: Blunt trauma to the head with or without subsequent skull fracture can cause the dura to separate from the inner table. As blood accumulates between the dura and the inner table, an epidural hematoma (EDH) is formed. The periosteal surface of the dura normally adheres densely to the inner table; this adherence prevents the formation of any epidural space. Separation of the dura from the inner table can occur ipsilateral or contralateral to the area of trauma. The source of bleeding into the epidural space can be the dural sinuses, the intradiploic veins, the meningeal vessels, or an injury to the middle meningeal artery or its anterior or posterior vessels. The classic CT scan of a brain with an epidural hematoma shows a sharply defined, high-attenuation density located between the inner table of the skull and the brain. The mass compresses the brain and can compress the ipsilateral-lateral ventricle, thereby resulting in a midline shift. Hematomas are restricted by sutural dural attachments.

Subdural hematoma: A serosanguineous collection occurring between the inner layer of the dura and the arachnoid, a subdural hematoma (SDH) is created when a subdural space is created by blood coming primarily from tears in the superficial cerebral cortical veins that separate the arachnoid and the dura. A SDH can occur on the side of impact, but it usually occurs on the opposite side; it follows ventricular depression of communicating hydrocephalus, with bleeding caused by the rapid stretching and disruption of veins already injured by posttraumatic SDH. Commonly located over the parietal cortical convexity, SDH can also be located above the tenorium cerebelli. The classic CT scan of acute SDH shows a crescent-shaped homogenous high-attenuation mass developing between the skull and the cerebral cortex but not including the sutural-dural limitation common with EDH.

Atypical subdural hematoma: Approximately 25% of acute subdural hematoma cases are atypical in that the hematoma is characterized as heterogenous and lentiform in configuration with minor convexities across the inner surface. Atypical subdural hematoma frequently results in a subsequent enlargement of the ipsilateral-lateral ventricle, which can be displaced across the midline. Atypical SDH can be caused by bleeding resulting from a coagulopathy with a low-intensity component that represents unclotted blood; by serum extruded during the early stages of clot retraction; or by CSF that enters from an arachnoid tear and mixes with blood. The temporal stages of bleeding further complicate the CT diagnosis of SDH, and subacute or chronic SDH can contain CT attenuation differences due to hematocrit effects.

Hematocrit effects can occur with atypical subdural hematoma (SDH) when the cellular elements maintain high CT attenuation and the serum maintains low CT attenuation in response to the traumatic event. This development could also result from rebleeding into an existing SDH. This phenomenon in CT can be misleading to practitioners who are unprepared for its possibility. Chronic SDH can be isodense as it relates to the adjacent cerebral cortex and can be recognized only by the displacement of the cortex, a midline shift, or ventricular compression. Isodense SDH can be more clearly visible on wide-window, or brain, CT images or with the use of an IV contrast agent.

Subarachnoid hemorrhage: Blood usually enters the subarachnoid space in response to trauma. A subarachnoid hemorrhage (SAH) results from disruption of the small vessels passing through the arachnoid space, direct tear of arteries and veins beneath a fracture or other penetrating traumatic event, or tears in cortical surface vessels. The usual scan of a brain with a SAH shows the blood at a high-attenuation density as it occurs in the sulci, the basilar cisterns, and the interpeduncular cistern with skull-base fractures. This blood causes the falx to cover the posterolateral surfaces of the sagittal sinus and to become dense with irregular margins. These changes result in a pseudo-delta sign, which indicates a filling defect in the sagittal sinus on the contrast-enhanced CT image of the head but resembles thrombosis in the sagittal sinus. On CT images obtained without contrast agents, the pseudo-delta sign is represented by the high intensity of the subarachnoid blood in the margins of the sagittal sinus and the low intensity of unenhanced sinus blood.

Diffuse brain edema: Diffuse brain edema is common in association with trauma and hypertension in adults and with child abuse, aspiration by pediatric patients, and strangulation. The CT scan shows diffuse cerebral edema, typically manifested by the effacement of the cortical sulci, the loss of the gray-white interface, and the compression of ventricles.

Diffuse axonal injury: Usually the result of acceleration-deceleration injury to the head, diffuse axonal injury (DAI), or white matter shear injury, can follow direct blunt trauma to the head when the speed of the movement of the brain lags behind the speed of the movement of the skull, thus tearing the axons at the junction of the gray and white matter. Most of the injury occurs deep to the cortex, and consequent CT scans typically show a small portion of the irregular, high-intensity signals in the periphery of the frontal lobes. DAI causes immediate, irreversible damage that can lead to severe posttraumatic dementia.

Intracerebral hemorrhage: An intracerebral hemorrhage is characterized by the introduction of and a subsequent increase in bleeding from the brain into the cerebral parenchyma. The most common causes of this nontraumatic occurrence of hemorrhaging include hypertension, vascular malformations, and cerebral aneurysms. The thalamus is a common site of damage caused by hypertension, a leading cause of intracerebral hemorrhaging in adults.

Almost 50% of hypertensive intracerebral hemorrhages require practitioners to perform a dissection into the ventricular system. On axial noncontrast CT scans, intracerebral hemorrhages can appear as an area of high attenuation in the cerebral parenchyma.

Hydrocephalus: An accumulation of excessive amounts of cerebrospinal fluid (CSF), hydrocephalus occurs in the ventricular system as the result of an impaired resorption or an obstruction in the flow of CSF that may either be communicating (i.e., nonobstructive) when the ventricular system is enlarged or noncommunicating (i.e., obstructive) when a portion of the ventricular system is affected. Ventricular and sulcal dilation occurs proportionally in brain atrophy, but hydrocephalus disproportionately enlarges the ventricles and not the sulci. CT scans show hydrocephalus within the temporal horns of the lateral ventricle, which indicates increased intraventricular pressure, with a width of almost 3 mm. The cortical sulci can become effaced with any marked or increasing intraventricular pressure.

Brain herniation: Brain herniation is the displacement of part of the brain as it is shifted in the skull through various openings in the inelastic dura as the result of diffuse or focal intracranial pressures. Subfalcine or cingulated herniation is a lateral herniation of the cingulated gyrus beneath the falx. Axial CT scans demonstrate herniation of the corpus callosum and the ipsilateral lateral ventricle under the falx. Rostrocaudal (transtentorial or downward) herniation can be lateral or central. Lateral herniation is characterized by the movement of medial portions of the temporal lobe, or uncus, through tentorial incisura. Uncal herniation is typified by compression of the ipsilateral ambient, or perimesencephalic, cistern and asymmetry of the 6-pointed suprasellar cistern when unilateral. Central transtentorial herniation is typified on axial CT because of massive cerebral edema or a large axial or extra-axial hemorrhage caused by severe compression of the suprasellar cistern, the fourth ventricle, and all cisterns around the midbrain.

Stroke: A cerebral infarction, or ischemic stroke, results in neurologic dysfunction and is the most common reason for admission to emergency departments or comparable facilities. Emboli are the most common cause of cerebral infarction and are most often associated with common carotid bifurcation and the internal carotid artery. The second most common cause of stroke is thrombosis of either the middle cerebral artery (MCA) or other major arteries. CT has become more essential in assessing patients with nontraumatic but persistent neurologic deficits because recent medical advances have produced systemic and local thrombolytic agents that can be initiated within a 1- to 5-hour window from the onset of the condition.

CT analysis after stroke: CT scans of the head can provide enough information about the condition of the brain at the time of the procedure to allow practitioners to rule out such conditions as intracranial hemorrhage, infection, or tumor as possible causes or origins of the neurologic signs and symptoms that would suggest the development of a stroke. However, head CT scans obtained within the first 6 hours of the onset of the ischemic stroke will appear normal; they will not demonstrate a neurologic deficit that the practitioner can recognize and diagnose accurately. Arterial embolism and thrombosis can be delineated more accurately by CT angiography. The earliest pathologic changes associated with brain infarction can be seen more easily with MRI and diffusion MRI, because these imaging methods are more suited than CT to this degree of specificity.

Noncontrast CT scans of the head taken soon after a brain infarction show 3 distinct developments in the brain: hyperdensity resulting from acute thrombus in the region of the anterior or middle cerebral artery; hypodensity in the basilar ganglia resulting in a loss of insular cortex; and hypodensity in the white matter resulting in a slight mass effect. Research has shown that only approximately 5% of studies involving cerebral infarcts can be described as initially hemorrhagic. A lacunar infarct is an occlusion of an end artery that supplies the deep gray and white matter, especially the area related to the basilar ganglia. On noncontrast CT these lacunar infarcts will most commonly appear in the basilar ganglia as small hypodense areas, because these infarcted areas become cystic.

Process of a stroke: During a stroke, the brain experiences a loss of blood supply and therefore cannot sustain healthy cells. This interruption of blood flow prevents oxygen and other important nutrients from being delivered throughout the brain and results in abnormal brain function. The blood flow to the brain can be disrupted by rupture or blockage of an artery that connects with the brain. A cerebral hemorrhage can occur when bleeding takes place within the brain substance, or a subarachnoid hemorrhage can occur when bleeding takes place between the inside of the skull and the brain itself. Arteries can become clogged within the brain, as with a lacunar stroke, or a carotid artery occlusion can occur in the arteries leading to the brain, whereupon those arteries harden. The heart and an artery can also pass an embolism to the brain, which will negatively affect normal brain function.

TIA: A transient ischemic attack occurs when a clot forms spontaneously within a blood vessel of the brain and causes a loss of blood supply to the brain that results in transient presenting symptoms and temporary effects on the patient. A TIA usually causes a loss of function in the area of the body controlled by the part of the brain affected. TIAs can also occur when clots that form in other parts of the body dislodge and travel as an embolus to an artery in the brain. Spasms and bleeding can cause TIAs, which are commonly referred to as mini-strokes. Although the effects of TIAs are noticeable only within 24 hours, the patient's condition should be analyzed immediately because TIAs can precede a permanent stroke and can leave sections of dead brain cells that would be noticeable on a CT scan.

Contrast media

CT is the procedure of choice for successful scanning examinations of most organs in the chest, abdomen, and pelvis. These scans can be performed with either enteric or intravenous contrast agents, although certain applications can be completed only without the use of contrast material, including evaluations for renal calculi and pulmonary nodules. Most abdominal and pelvic scans, excluding renal stone examinations, require the administration of intravenous or oral contrast material for the production of improved images to be used for evaluating the condition of these areas. The female reproductive tract and the gallbladder do not respond as well to CT contrast materials as they do to ultrasonography. However, CT scanning provides remarkable visualization of other internal organs, such as the liver, spleen, kidneys, intestines, pancreas, and retroperitoneal structures.

How contrast materials work

The contrast materials used during CT provide a clearer outline of the organs and tissues being studied, thereby allowing the practitioner to differentiate between body parts for analysis. CT scans are usually taken before the contrast agent is administered and then again after the contrast agent has been administered. This procedure clarifies the structures being studied. The x-rays penetrate body parts differently in response to the types of tissue present. Bone appears white on CT scans, whereas air appears black. The densities of the various tissues are assigned values or density coefficients, and the computer can calculate these values to produce a three-dimensional representation of the body for display on a computer monitor. Practitioners can choose a particular section or slice of the body for additional study, and those images can be printed for further research.

Indications

CT allows practitioners to determine visually whether a growth or development is benign or malignant; such a determination is based on the image densities. CT is also used to diagnose such conditions as stroke, bleeding, injuries, tumors, abscesses, cysts, swelling or inflammation, blood or fluid accumulation, anatomic abnormalities, perforation, obstruction, aneurysms, and kidney stones or other types of stones.

Contraindications:

Not all patients can undergo CT because of contraindications, including pregnancy, obesity, or severe claustrophobia. Patients whose vital signs are unstable also cannot undergo CT. Patients should be asked about such contraindications and about any allergic reactions to materials as iodine or shellfish. Allergic reactions may not rule out CT scanning but may affect the choice of contrast agent.

Dose calculation:

Most practitioners refer to a CT dose-calculation program when selecting the appropriate radiation dosage for a patient undergoing CT. The dose-length product is currently regarded as the reference dose descriptor for these patients, although determining the effective dose is necessary for estimating the risk to the patient that may occur from any given CT procedure. Such risks are not addressed by the dose-length product. The CT dose-calculation program uses a Monte Carlo simulation routine to estimate the dose distribution and the effective dose through mathematically described phantoms associated with a particular CT protocol, scanner type, and dose-length product. The CT dose-calculation program is the preferred method for showing the consequences of scanning border and target regions, estimating the dose level for the protocol, estimating population doses, and establishing conversion factors between dose-length product and effective dose.

Scanning procedures

Positioning

Even the most sensitive CT equipment cannot provide practitioners with accurate images if the patient or couch moves during testing. Most CT scans must be repeated if the patient moves at all, because such movement affects the entire sequencing of the machine and provides skewed images for analysis. Most health care facilities provide cushions and other articles to make the patient as comfortable as possible without changing positions during the test. Some type of physical restraint or support cushion can be given to the patient for maintaining the proper positioning of the skull and alleviating the tension that occurs in the lower legs upon lying flat for a prolonged period of time. Proper CT positioning can result in improved success rates of detecting puncture foramen ovale and in decreased complication rates associated with the testing. CT positioning is more consistent than traditional positioning, and its clinical application is better.

Spiral CT

Older, more conventional CT has been replaced in many health care facilities by spiral or helical CT, which is a similar procedure used to image the head, abdomen, and chest. Spiral CT, however, provides faster image acquisition and improved 3D imaging. The efficient speed of spiral CT is often advantageous for patients who are claustrophobic or cannot remain still for long periods of time. The contrast can be followed more quickly, and the patient dose can be reduced so that the pitch is greater than 1. No misregistration is noted, and the patient can enjoy an increased throughput and comfort level. CT angiography (CTA) incorporates spiral CT technology with contrast agents to assist practitioners in studying blood vessels with fewer motion and partial-volume artifacts.

Longer processing time: Although spiral CT has replaced conventional CT in most facilities, spiral CT requires more time for image processing because the higher amount of information gathered by spiral CT requires interpolation before planar image reconstruction is performed. Spiral CT overlooks no anatomy in the scanned volume and can be reconstructed at any z-axis position. Image noise is normally less with spiral CT, and practitioners can attain multiple overlapping transverse images during a single breathhold by the patient without any additional patient dose. The z-axis resolution is slightly compromised in spiral CT, although practitioners can reconstruct images and better detect small lesions.

Reconstruction: Spiral CT has been shown to significantly improve coronal and sagittal slice reconstruction by creating high-quality 2D and 3D image reformations through overlapping transverse images. The interval at which the images can be reconstructed is called the index, which is often defined as the reconstruction distance divided by the collimation. An index less than 1 indicates image overlap, whereas an index greater than 1 indicates a gap. Practitioners can use an index of less than 1 when attempting to visualize suspected lung nodules. Scan time, beam collimation, couch feed velocity, and z-axis spacing for image reconstruction are unique components of each spiral CT scan, and the computer memory must be extensive because the images are acquired faster than they are reconstructed. The scan time must not exceed 25 s, the normal length of a patient's breathhold.

Interpolation: Interpolation is the computation of unknown values by using known values on either side. Conventional CT can produce only contiguous reconstruction, resulting in partial-volume effect when the object is contained in adjacent slices of equal thickness. Spiral CT provides the practitioner with the ability to overlap the reconstructive portion, making it possible to ensure that an observed object is fully contained within a slice. The data acquired by spiral CT is continuous along the z-axis, so that image reconstruction can be completed at any z-axis position through interpolation. Collimation determines the slice thickness and is not contingent on the z-axis position, and volume averaging increases as pitch increases.

Spiral CT of the head and neck: Standard spiral CT of the head and neck comprises several similar elements. Unlike spiral CT of the chest, the results of spiral CT of the head and neck are less subject to differentiation caused by respiratory motion. The slice thickness is normally 2.5 mm, whereas the slice thickness for spiral CT of the chest is typically 10 mm. In spiral CT of the head and neck, the couch movement is normally 1.5 mm/s; in spiral CT of the chest, the couch movement is 15-20 mm/s. The imaging portion of spiral CT begins 50 seconds after the bolus injection. Although practitioners may differ in their choice of contrast agent, most agree that approximately 100 mL of the contrast agent should be injected at 1-2 mL/s.

Dynamic CT

Dynamic CT involves dynamic scanning, which consists of 15 or more scans completed in rapid succession within a minute. This procedure can be used for such specialized evaluations as trauma, cardiac, and vascular imaging. Dynamic CT allows the practitioner to image arteries immediately after a bolus injection. Although dynamic scanning typically involves 15 one-second scans, each of those 15 scans is divided by a defined 2-second interscan time so that the couch can be adjusted to a distance equivalent to the slice thickness. This type of scan has specialized limitations, including the required time for tube cooling, which has greatly limited the extent of dynamic scanning. Because of these insurmountable limitations, most practitioners use spiral CT.

Multislice imaging

First produced by Elscint and now available from all CT manufacturers, multislice imaging (MI) involves the use of 2 or more contiguous detector arrays and produces 2 or more section images at the same time. As a spiral CT technique, MI is responsible for greatly reducing imaging time from about 3 minutes with conventional CT to less than 30 seconds with spiral CT. Although the main advantage of MI is faster imaging capabilities with better spatial resolution, MI requires an exceptional engineering basis because of the mechanical forces that are produced by the gantry rotation. The complete rotation of the x-ray tube and detector array takes less than 1 second, whereas partial scan images are available within approximately 100 ms. The best imaging requires a pitch of about 3:1 to 6:1.

Interpolation: The image reconstruction involved in multislice imaging (MI) incorporates 360° interpolation instead of the standard 180°. This interpolation allows for faster imaging combined with noise reduction and an improved spatial and temporal resolution of the multislice images. The faster couch speed also provides for a reduction in misregistration of anatomy, and motional artifacts are subsequently also reduced. MI offers patients a less-demanding breathhold while imaging a larger z-axis volume in less time. Practitioners can administer smaller amounts of contrast material, and the patient has an increased throughput. Post-processing in MI allows for variable slice thickness and fewer requirements for rescanning. Practitioners have found that CTA is greatly improved when MI is included, and many have found that coronary artery calcification assay with MI is challenging with regard to electron beam CT (EBCT).

MDCT

A form of interventional neuroradiology, multidetector helical CT-guided spine intervention (MDCT) allows CT scanning of patients with implanted metal hardware because of previous trauma or surgical procedures. This complex spine imaging procedure allows practitioners obtain CT images of patients who have extensive spinal hardware; the image is not marred by metal artifact. Such images allow practitioners to study the hardware itself and to determine whether follow-up interventions are necessary. Research is ongoing to improve this type of real-time, image-guided therapy. Once the z-axis coverage can be increased, practitioners will be able to provide guidance by using MDCT in combination with x-ray fluoroscopy and CT system analysis, which will reduce the costs associated with these tests.

Evaluating coronary arteries: Multidetector CT is being used in combination with electron-beam CT (EBCT) to evaluate coronary arteries. This combination allows practitioners to detect and quantify arterial calcification, which indicates atherosclerosis and can lead to serious coronary risk in the future. CT can detect this calcification at an earlier stage than stress tests, which can detect stenosis of 50% or more. By comparing repeated measurements with a baseline measurement, practitioners can determine the progression of the disease and determine whether recommendations for diet and medication are appropriate for reducing the cardiac event. Prospective cardiac gating facilitates MDCT for evaluating coronary arteries with an inherent higher spatial resolution and increased detection of minute calcification.

Special procedures

Biopsies

Mediastinal biopsy: Practitioners can perform CT-guided lung biopsies in the standard fashion and review the relevant films before performing the actual procedure, which is the responsibility of the fellow or attending medical personnel. Patients with lung lesions may also have other intra-abdominal lesions, including adrenal masses, which are often easier to handle with image-guided biopsies because these biopsies are associated with fewer complications. The practitioner may review older images that show the lesion as benign and stable and determine that a biopsy is not appropriate. The booking radiologist should attempt to gather as much information as possible, even though the fellow or attending medical personnel are expected and required to perform the biopsy in the most appropriate area for the patient.

Renal biopsies for benign disease: An 18-gauge biopsy needle, or biopsy gun, is required for renal biopsies for benign disease, and the biopsy is still considered high-risk. Patients are admitted to the hospital on the day of the biopsy and must not be actively following an aspirin regimen before the procedure. Blood work is mandatory and must include typing and cross-matching. Completion of a prebiopsy form is usually required by the Quality Assurance Committee; this form must be attached to the medical record. Most medical facilities also require completion of a postbiopsy form endorsed by the Quality Assurance Committee; this form must be completed before the patient leaves the department and must be attached to the medical record. Renal biopsies for benign disease are usually performed under ultrasonographic guidance.

Renal biopsies for renal mass: Because admission to the hospital is not necessary for the completion of renal biopsy for a renal mass, the procedure can be performed on an outpatient basis. Most medical facilities handle renal biopsy for renal mass similarly to the way in which they handle liver biopsy. All biopsy examinations require completion of appropriate laboratory studies, such as determination of PT, PTT, INR, platelet count, hematocrit, hemoglobin concentration, and documented bleeding time. This detailed information assists the practitioner who will be completing the biopsy and who will be evaluating the results once the procedure is concluded. The prebiopsy and postbiopsy forms are required according to the facilities' regulations, and an intravenous line must be placed before the procedure. No work can be completed without the required documents and test completions.

Radiation therapy planning

The accuracy of imaging for radiation therapy treatment planning can be improved by the concurrent use of positron emission tomography and computed tomography (PET/CT). This combination of studies reduces the errors caused by organ motion and eliminates the waiting period required for completing CT in one department on one day and completing PET in another department on a different day before practitioners can analyze the results and diagnose the condition. Patients are often unable to maintain identical body positions after that much time between testing, and internal organs move and deform to different shapes, especially in reference to the variable filling volumes of the bladder and bowel. CT scans obtained during PET scanning are more accurate, and practitioners can better target cancer cells and deliver higher radiation doses to the foreign body with consideration made for normal tissue. This approach is associated with fewer side effects and more-effective treatments.

Drainage and aspiration

Processes such as abscess draining usually require antibiotic coverage. However, if antibiotics cannot be administered until after the specimen has been aspirated, they must be initiated immediately after the procedure has been completed. The Infectious Diseases Division recommends the intravenous administration of Unasyn (3 g) for broad-spectrum coverage after procedures for draining abdominal abscesses. Alternatively, Ancef (1 g) and gentamicin (80 g) may be given though the IV at the time of the procedure. Patients undergoing an abscess drainage procedure are generally admitted for overnight observation because all patients experience transient bacteremia and an episode of hypotension after the procedure.

CT angiography

Cerebral angiography: Also known as carotid angiography, cerebral angiography can confirm the occurrence of a stroke, especially if the patient is still within the window of opportunity for applying the appropriate medication to dissolve the clot. Cerebral angiography can also detect bulging of the arterial walls, blood clots, and arterial narrowing, or stenosis. Cerebral angiography can assist the practitioner in evaluating the arteries of the patient's head and neck before performing corrective surgery or in response to severe cases of head or neck trauma. Cerebral angiography is most often used to obtain more accurate information after MRI or CT of the head that shows an abnormal development or condition.

Aortic angiography: Aortic angiography studies the aorta, the large artery that distributes blood from the heart to various other arteries located throughout the body. Aortic angiography involves injecting contrast material through a catheter, a thin and flexible tube that has been placed in a strategic location. CT allows the catheter to be used as an IV site, usually in the arm, for administration of the contrast agent. This contrast material is visible on x-ray images and can demonstrate blockages or abnormal rates of blood flow through the aorta.

Procedure: A light sedative is administered to the patient before testing. An intravenous catheter is placed in the arm so that medication can be administered during the course of the procedure. A separate catheter can be placed in the patient's arm or groin through a small incision in an artery in the selected location. No incision is made until after the site has been cleansed and numbed with a local anesthetic. Fluoroscopy is used to guide the insertion of the catheter as it is carefully threaded into the aorta from the injection site in the arm or groin. Once the catheter is in place inside the aorta, the contrast dye is injected so that the aorta can be viewed. CT fluoroscopy involves high radiation doses to the patient and personnel.

Patient preparation: The patient will be advised to consume no food or drink for 6 to 8 hours before testing. Some practitioners require the patient be hospitalized on the night before the test, whereas other practitioners perform the procedure as either an outpatient or an inpatient procedure. Before the anesthetic is administered, the procedure and its associated risks will be explained to the patient, and the patient or the appropriate representative must sign the consent form. A mild sedative will be administered approximately 30 minutes before the procedure, and the effects of the sedative may persist for hours after the testing. All patients must wear hospital clothing, and practitioners will advise patients to have someone at the medical facility who can provide transportation once the procedure is finished.

Physics and Instrumentation

System Principles, Operation and Components

CT imagers

First-generation CT imagers

First-generation CT imagers combine the finely collimated, or restricted, x-ray or pencil beam with the fan-shaped x-ray or fan beam to focus on a single radiation detector. The machine completes a translate-rotate motion: 180 separate translations are completed at each degree and a single image projection for each completed translation. The image time is 5 minutes, and the imager can image the head only.

Second-generation CT imagers

Second-generation CT imagers use a fan beam but have multiple radiation detectors, or a detector array. The same translate-rotate motion is used but with 18 separate translations at each tenth degree and with multiple image projections for each completed translation. The image time is approximately 30 seconds, and the imager can image the head and the body.

Third-generation CT imagers

Third-generation CT imagers use a fan beam x-ray source to view the entire patient, not just the head or a particular portion of the body. The curvilinear detector array completes several hundred radiation detectors and maintains a constant distance between the source and each detector. This consistency results in good image reconstruction. The x-ray source and the detector array move about the same axis, and the rotate-rotate motion allows for 360° viewing. Each rotation provides hundreds of image projections with better spatial and contrast resolution, whereas different arc scans are used to improve motion blur for half or full scans. The image time is one second or less, but characteristic ring artifacts are present.

Fourth-generation CT imagers

Developed to suppress the occurrence of ring artifacts, fourth-generation CT imagers have an x-ray source collimated to a fan beam with a detector array containing several thousand individual detectors. The rotating motion of the x-ray source mechanism is rotate-stationary around the fixed detector array with the unattenuated leading and trailing edge of the fan beam to allow for individual detector calibration for each completed scan. The radiation dose to the patient is higher because of the interspace between detectors; x-radiation falls on the interspace and results in a wasted dose. The image projection is acquired as the fan beam passes across each detector and usually occurs in less than one second. Half-, full-, and over-arc scans are available.

Electron beam CT

Specifically developed for fast imaging, electron beam computed tomography (EBCT) obtains images in less than 100 ms, approximately the time required for obtaining a radiograph. A microwave-accelerated electron beam incident on a tungsten target is the x-ray source for EBCT; the target covers half of the imaging circle, and the detector array covers the other half. The curved tungsten target creates a moving source for the electron beam, and 4 contiguous images are created simultaneously by 4 targets, or focal tracks, and 4 detector arrays. With no moving parts, EBCT is principally associated with heart scanning in cardiac imaging.

<u>Spiral CT</u>

Currently the standard CT imaging method, spiral CT resulted from the development of slip rings, which allowed for data transfer from a rotating gantry. Able to image large volumes of body parts in less time, spiral CT scan image the entire torso during a single patient breathhold.

Components of a CT imager

All CT imagers consist of an operating console, a computer, and a gantry. Imaging control, with preselected technique conditions and image viewing and manipulation, is completed by the operating console, although several operating consoles may be attached to the CT to address various functions of the test, such as image analysis and CT control or post-processing. The computer itself has no identifiable CT features but must have a high capacity and must be very fast to handle the large number of computations that are required in an extensive data set. Any computer that is capable of multiprocessing can be used in CT. The gantry houses the x-ray source, the detector array, the collimator assembly, and the high-voltage generator if applicable. With the ability to tilt approximately 30° either way, the gantry has a patient aperture of approximately 70 cm as its maximum diameter.

<u>X-ray source</u>

The x-ray tube is designed to handle high x-ray intensity and rapid heat dissipation. The high intensity is reached with a high mA generator and a focal spot size of about 2 mm. Large-diameter, thick anode disks rotate at 10,000 RPM to provide rapid heat dissipation, although CT x-ray tubes were developed with a high heat capacity. The anode heat capacity commonly reaches 6 MHU (million heat units), whereas general radiography reaches less than 1 MHU. The x-ray tubes themselves have a high-speed rotor that maintains 10,000 RPM, and the anode-cathode axis is situated perpendicular to the patient axis in an effort to avoid the heel effect, whereby x-rays are absorbed in the heel of the target. This heel effect could cause reduced x-ray intensity on the anode side of the central axis.

<u>Slip rings</u>

Found in some CT scanners, slip rings are the mechanisms that facilitate the continuous rotation of the x-ray tube by replacing cables. Slip rings function to conduct power and electrical signals to various points throughout the gantry. Using circular electrical conductors, slip rings rotate and pass power to the high-voltage generator and also pass signals from the data acquisition system (DAS) to the computer. The DAS also converts an analog signal to digital (ADC) and amplifies the detector signal. The technology designed for use with slip rings provides continuous data acquisition and a capability for faster imaging that can be attained without interscan delay, cable wrap, or start-stop motions. Slip rings permit the connection between the x-ray source and the high-frequency generator located at the fixed part of the gantry.

Generator and transformers

<u>High-voltage generator</u>

Patient dose can be reduced by high kVp, which also minimizes the photoelectric absorption. Bone attenuation can be reduced by high kVp as it relates to soft tissue that allows a wider dynamic range of the image. Radiation intensity can be increased at the detector array with high kVp, and the tube life can be extended and the x-ray tube loading reduced with high kVp and lower mA. Also called three-phase generators, high-frequency voltage generators consist of three-phase voltage, which is usually generated by a stand-alone module next to the gantry. A reversal of gantry rotation can be accomplished because of the cables of the high-voltage generator that can wind 360°. The generators themselves are small enough to be mounted on the rotating gantry, whereas slip rings make continuous rotation of the x-ray source possible and allows spiral CT.

Detector

Detector array

A grouping of detectors, the detector array has improved continually during the course of the CT evolution, and the efficiency of its use has determined the maximum tube loading and has controlled the subsequent patient dose. Healthcare facilities use both gas-filled and solid-state detector arrays. Gas-filled detectors have about 50% detection efficiency with fast response and no afterglow. Using high-pressure gas, gas-filled detectors can be packed more tightly than solid-state detectors and use less interspace septa. The gas-filled detector has small ion chambers, each about 1 mm wide, that can be filled with xenon or another comparable gas that handles pressure well. Solid-state detectors use a cadmium tungstate ($CdWO_4$) scintillator that is optically coupled to a photodiode. With nearly 100% detection efficiency, solid-state detectors cannot be tightly packed. The detector array is geometrically efficient with a 90% detector area and little interspace.

Detection efficiency: Multiplying the geometric efficiency of the detector array by the intrinsic efficiency yields the total detector efficiency, which depends on the number of detectors and the tightness of their packing. Solid-state detectors commonly produce 80% total detection efficiency. With solid-state detectors, all incident x-rays are detected because of the 90% intrinsic efficiency of the device. Made of a scintillation crystal, solid-state detectors emit light that is converted into an analog signal by the photodiode when the crystal is irradiated. Any space between detectors reduces the detection efficiency and increases the patient dose. Automatically recalibrated between scans, a solid-state detector is more expensive than a gas-filled detector, but the increased efficiency could result in less x-ray tube loading, reduced patient dose, and reduced image noise.

Collimation

Multi-detector CT (MDCT) allows practitioners to access, process, and display the appropriate parameters of a patient's body sections through CT and computer-aided detection (CAD) with great room for further development. Practitioners have achieved better success by using a narrower collimation and thin reconstructions in MDCT to realize a higher accuracy level when using a CAD algorithm. The accuracy of that algorithm can be highly dependent on reconstruction thickness, although this dependence is not well documented in the associated imaging literature or the practice guidelines for CAD image acquisition. Healthcare facilities that rely on CAD programs for MDCT scans should consider that the sensitivity of the program might be higher with the reconfigured collimation limits and subsequent slices.

CT computer

The CT computer consists of an input device, a CPU, an output device, and memory, because the CT computer must have exceptional memory capabilities so that it can manipulate the extensive amounts of data that are obtained through even simple CT scans. The input/output (I/O) devices of the CT computer are used as supplementary pieces of computer hardware that have been designed to place raw data into the computer and to receive processed data from the computer. Input devices include the keyboard, tape, disk, video display terminal, CT detector, CD-ROM, plasma screen, and laser screen. Output devices include the laser camera, dry image processor, video display terminal, printer, and image transmitter. The CPU houses the control unit, primary memory, and the microprocessor and acts as the brains of the machine.

Components

Designed as a computer on a chip or a wafer, the microprocessor is made of silicon that has been fabricated into many transistors and diodes and that works with the control unit and memory to provide consistency and accuracy from the CPU. The control unit runs the computer functions while also interpreting instructions and sequencing tasks. The primary memory can be located either on the CPU or on an additional circuit board and can exist as read-only memory (ROM), random-access memory (RAM), or write-one-time, read-many-times (WORM) memory for storing data used in the various computations completed by the computer. This memory is solid state and can be made of silicon or semiconductor technology, providing very fast components that are limited in size.

Secondary memory: CT computers use secondary memory functions whenever the primary memory is insufficient or the data must be transferred to another location. Useful for the bulk storage of various types of information, including images of differing memory sizes, secondary memory can be configured as "all online" by using magnetic hard drive disks or as "all offline" by using magnetic tape and magnetic or optical disks. Software is an important resource for secondary memory functions of the CT computer because the collections of software programs are written in computer language and can implement the numerous tasks completed by the computer, such as look-up tables (LUT). All computers use operating systems software, such as Microsoft Windows, DOS, and UNIX, to manage the computer hardware, whereas application programs are written in a higher-level language and include the necessary algorithms for image reconstruction and post-processing analysis.

Array processor

A special type of computer, the analog-to-digital converter (ADC), converts the analog signal from each CT detector into a digital form that the computer can manipulate during imaging. Another special type of computer, the array processor, is designed to handle single tasks, such as image reconstruction, quickly and accurately. The main CT computer itself must have the capacity to solve a large numbers of equations concurrently so that the system can produce a 512 x 512 matrix, which means that the computer must be able to solve 262,144 equations simultaneously. Multiple microprocessors contribute to the accomplishment of most of the CT computer functions, although most image reconstructions are performed by the array processor. The reconstruction time consists of the interval between the end of imaging or data collection and the final manipulation or appearance of the image; most systems commonly produce images at 1 s or less.

CTAs

CTA is noninvasive and the examination can be completed within seconds. Practitioners can use aneurysm clips and can analyze the lumen and vessel walls through multiplanar imaging. The process itself can be performed emergently with the administration of 15 cc or less of a central contrast agent. CTA is traditionally less expensive and involves a lower radiation dose than conventional angiography. However, CTA also has limitations. CTA depends on specific software and hardware, and postprocessing may require a separate work station. CTA produces classic CT artifacts and presents its best spatial resolution at 0.3 mm or 21 p/cm.

Quantitative computed tomography

Using a region of interest (ROI) to determine the average CT number of a tissue for potential use as an aid to the practitioner in diagnosis, quantitative computed tomography (QCT) can greatly assist practitioners in identifying and characterizing a tumor by differentiating between solid and cystic lesions in the body. QCT is effective in determining measurements of density and in characterizing the structure of lung tissue by incorporating spirometric control and breath-triggered imaging. QCT allows practitioners to measure cerebral blood flow in patients who have inhaled xenon gases and also provides assistance in measuring tissue perfusion in patients after a bolus injection of an iodinated contrast agent.

Hounsfield Units and attenuation coefficients

At 125 kVp, dense bone measures at 1000 HU with a μ of 0.4600, whereas muscle measures at 50 HU with a μ of 0.2310. White matter and gray matter are closely related at 125 kVp: white matter measures at 45 HU with a μ of 0.1870, and gray matter measures at 40 HU with a μ of 0.1840. Interestingly, blood and cerebrospinal fluid are also closely aligned: blood measures at 20 HU with a μ of 0.1820, and cerebrospinal fluid measures at 15 HU with a μ of 0.1810. At 125 kVp water measures at 0 HU with a μ of 0.1800. Fat and lungs measure more widely than other tissues: fat measures at –100 HU with a μ of 0.1620, and lungs measure at –200 HU with a μ of 0.0940. Air is at the lower extreme: it measures at –1000 HU with a μ of 0.0003.

Sensitivity

Sensitivity is the ability of the digital image receptor to respond to the x-rays being passed over the body part being studied. Because practitioners want to expose CT patients to the least amount of radiation possible, they focus on realizing the most sufficient minimum signal detected by the machinery with the best potential for review and study.

Spatial frequency

Spatial frequency is used to express size by measuring changes in the tissue attenuation characteristics of different organs and tissues within the body. Any defined changes in the tissue, as exhibited by movement from rib bones to air sacs in the lungs, will show a high spatial frequency, whereas gradual changes, as exhibited by movement from the liver to the spleen, will show a low spatial frequency. This measurement is described in line pair per millimeter, or lp/mm.

Resolution

Resolution provides the ability to distinguish between similar types of tissues on the CT image, such as gray and white matter in the brain, or the liver and the spleen. CT imaging handles contrast resolution better than any other facet of image quality. The contrast resolution completed with x-ray imaging is determined by the atomic number of the tissue (Z), the mass density ρ (kg/m^3), and the electron density (e/m^3). Tissues that differ greatly in Z and ρ will produce a high level of contrast on CT images. Contrast resolution is improved during radiographic imaging, whereas scatter radiation and kVp are reduced. This fact is important because CT uses high kVp to minimize the radiation dose to the patient.

Image Processing and Display

Image reconstruction

CT imaging extrapolates information from data acquisition, image display, and image reconstruction. Preprocessing, or the reformatting and convolution of the image, occurs between data acquisition and image reconstruction. Post-processing, recording, and archiving follow the image display. Using a keyboard and a disk as input devices, image reconstruction involves the review of filtered back image projection that results in a digital matrix. This digital matrix can be post-processed for additional image analysis. Each pixel received is computed and is assigned a CT number. The sagittal image crosses the body lengthwise along the nose, whereas the coronal image crosses the body lengthwise along the side of the head and the transverse image crosses the body widthwise just under the nose.

Filtered back-projection reconstruction

For optimal computer operation, the environment of the laboratory should be consistently maintained at less than 30% relative humidity with a temperature below 20°C (70°F). Under optimal conditions, the detector element records the analog image projection so that the DAS can transfer that information to the ADC. The ADC converts the image to a digital image projection, and each digital image projection acquired by individual detectors can be stored in the computer's memory. Convoluted back projection reconstructs the CT images from the image projections by using simultaneous filtered back projection of all image projections. Back-projection is a reconstruction algorithm applied to CT in a set of well-defined computer software sequences that has been designed to produce an image, or output, from a signal profile, or input.

Interaction between filters and back-projection: CT scanning widely uses back-projection with a convolution filter, or filtered back-projection, so that the convolution filters can produce volume- and surface-rendered images. The convolution filter is not made of aluminum or copper, nor is it used to reduce or deflect low-energy x-ray beams. In CT, the convolution filter mathematically manipulates specific data to change the appearance of the image. Sometimes called a kernel, the convolution filter applies a mathematical process to an image projection before back-projection occurs. Both convolution filters and reconstructive algorithms can suppress high-frequency signals when they are configured for high frequency. The higher frequency causes the image to appear smooth and may improve contrast resolution.

Image clarity: On its own, back-projection can result in a blurred image because the x-ray attenuation is not uniform over the entire path length of the image. Convolution filters can correct projection angulation because this angulation commonly results in blurred images. Practitioners use a convolution filter with back-projection so that the image projections that are visible before reconstruction can be sharper and more accurate, thereby leading to less error on the part of the practitioner. Although high-frequency convolution filters can produce smoother images, a low-frequency convolution filter can suppress low-frequency signals so that the edge is enhanced and the spatial resolution can possibly be improved. Although the image projections are overlapped, most CT imagers have more than 20 available convolution filters so that the practitioner can select the quality of the image.

Reconstruction filters

Practitioners can request images with enhanced contrast resolution or enhanced spatial resolution. Spatial frequency is determined by how rapidly the subject contrast changes; the interface of bone and soft tissue exhibits high spatial frequency because the object is small and the contrast is high; in contrast, the interface of gray matter and white matter in the brain exhibits low spatial frequency because the object is large and the contrast is low. Using an appropriate convolution filter can enhance or suppress the spatial frequencies of the various tissues imaged. For bone and inner ear images, high-pass convolution filters suppress low spatial frequencies and enhance high spatial frequencies, thereby producing images with enhanced edges, more noise, and a short contrast scale. For brain and liver images, low-pass convolution filters suppress high spatial frequencies and enhance low spatial frequencies, thereby producing images with less noise and a long contrast scale. Image reconstruction time is determined by the convolution filter, the ADC rate, the data, and the CPU clock speed.

Raw data vs. image data

Slice images and masks are types of data used in 3D reconstructions. Slice images consist of a sequence of sections through the body part or object of interest and can be obtained directly through mechanical slicing or through tomographic reconstruction. Masks provide a geometric representation of the particular body parts or objects of interest and can be obtained through manual or image-processing segmentation of the images. Raw data shown in a slice image consist of each pixel that has an unsigned byte, whereas image data include scan lines that are stored by rows. Each dataset includes information about the number and size of the images. CT data may consist of axial CT scans of the head and neck taken at 1-mm intervals at a resolution of 512 x 512 pixels with each pixel defined by 24 bits of color, or approximately 7.5 Mb.

Effective slice thickness

The transition from axial to helical to multi-detector helical scanning produces some concern about reconstructed slice thickness and about how an effective slice thickness will change between tests, even when the same patient is undergoing the test. The factors that could influence slice thickness include x-ray beam collimation, especially in single-slice CT scanners; detector width, especially in MDCT; helical pitch or table speed; and helical interpolation algorithm. Reconstructed slice thickness is considered independently in some MDCT scanners because the interpolation algorithm is used. Under these conditions, the pitch or table speed would be closely linked to the interpolation algorithm. Higher table speeds produce large effective slice thicknesses in single-detector helical scanners, whereas the table speed in multi-detector scanners can affect slice thickness and the sensitivity profile.

Importance: Practitioners who image CT scans in different parts of the body notice a difference in the resulting image and the subsequent slice thickness used to obtain that image. CT scans that focus on the patient's chest can usually be completed by using a standard or high-resolution protocol. Obtaining such images would require very thin slices (approximately 1 mm thick) in high-resolution chest scanning evaluations obtained at 10-mm intervals through the chest region. Normally, this same type of scan is acquired and displayed only in bone or lung algorithms, which facilitate the evaluation of lung parenchyma. This type of study is useful for evaluating interstitial lung disease. Pelvic fractures, however, can be better evaluated with both sagittal and coronal reformations with the acquisition of three-dimensional volume-rendering images. These images assist the practitioner in the repair of the fracture.

Image display

All CT images are formatted as a matrix with digital properties. The matrix is an organized array of cells; the cells, or pixels, are arranged in columns and rows to create a digital image. The matrix used in current CT imagers can produce images with a resolution of 512 x 512 pixels; however, many CT imagers can produce images with a resolution of 1024 x 1024 pixels, and the larger matrix size produces better spatial resolution, although a longer reconstruction time is necessary. A CT imager capable of producing images with a resolution of 1024 x 1024 pixels computes 1,048,576 simultaneous equations into 1,048,576 matrix cells. Each cell is a picture element, or pixel, and presents a two-dimensional representation of a volume element, or voxel. The voxel size is determined by the combination of the pixel size and the section thickness.

The principal cause of CT imager malfunction is a failure in the x-ray tube. Currents in the x-ray tube commonly range from 200 to 800 mA. When the mA is too low, unacceptable image noise results. The usual x-ray tube potential ranges from 120 kVp to 140 kVp three phase or high frequency, although high kVp is used with higher intensity and penetrability, which results in less x-ray tube loading and lower patient dose. Dual-focus tubes are common in the x-ray source, with typical 0.5- to 1.0-mm focal spots, which can be used to produce better spatial resolution. The better x-ray beam or radiation detector collimation will result in improved spatial resolution, although matrix size and field of view (FOV) produce the principal effect on spatial resolution.

Pixel

A pixel is a picture element found in a digital image and is categorized by a CT number for the purposes of image display. Pixels are also important components of a digital image matrix.

Voxel

A voxel is a volume element as the most basic element used to define the volume of tissue represented by each pixel in a reconstructed image.

Matrix

A matrix is an array of numbers found in rows and columns of pixels that are displayed in a digital image and are usually written as N x N. Although the number of pixels in an image defines the size of the matrix, the matrix size and the FOV determine the spatial resolution of the image. A larger matrix size, e.g., 1024 x 1024 instead of 512 x 512, will result in smaller pixels and provide better spatial resolution. Smaller matrix sizes are commonly used in pediatric imaging and biopsy localization because in such cases spatial resolution is not as important as contrast resolution. A normally scanned FOV averages approximately 20 cm for the head or pediatric body, 35 cm for the body, and 48 cm for a large body. Practitioners can use the localizer images when determining the extent of the anatomy to be imaged. These localizer images are also digital radiographic images and are made while the patient couch moves through the beam.

Relationship with FOV and pixel size: Pixel size is determined by the size of the matrix and the field of view (FOV). A matrix size of 512 x 512 with an FOV of 12 cm will produce a pixel size of 0.23 mm. A matrix size of 512 x 512 with an FOV of 30 cm, however, will produce a pixel size of 0.59 mm. Larger matrix sizes result in smaller pixel sizes when the FOV is held constant. A matrix size of 1024 x 1024 with an FOV of 12 cm will produce a pixel size of 0.12 mm. A matrix size of 1024 x 1024 with an FOV of 30 cm, however, will produce a pixel size of 0.29 mm. Larger FOV results in larger pixel sizes when the matrix size is held constant.

Field of view

The field of view (FOV) is the diameter of the reconstructed image. When the FOV is increased while the matrix size is held constant, the pixel size is increased and the spatial resolution is reduced. Smaller pixel sizes can be attained only by decreasing the FOV or by increasing the matrix size. When the matrix size is increased while the FOV is held constant, the pixel size is reduced and the spatial resolution is improved. Generally, the pixel size limits the spatial resolution of the CT imager. Images creased with smaller pixels exhibit better spatial resolution and contain high-frequency information, whereas images created with larger pixels exhibit reduced spatial resolution and contain low-frequency information.

Scanned field of view and displayed field of view: The scanned field of view can be equal to or greater than the displayed field of view. The scanned field of view (SFOV) is usually configured to cover the anatomic part of the patient, commonly referred to as the head, body, or large body. The displayed field of view (DFOV), however, is most often used during the post-processing portion of the imaging to provide the practitioner with a magnified image of a portion of the SFOV. When practitioners employ magnification in either the SFOV or the DFOV by using the original image projections, or target zoom, the spatial resolution improves. When practitioners employ an easier and faster magnification in either the SFOV or the DFOV by using pixel enlargement, or photo zoom, the spatial resolution decreases.

CT numbers

CT numbers refer to those numbers used to define the relative attenuation coefficient for each pixel of studied tissue in an image in comparison to the attenuation coefficient of water. A numerical value, or CT number, is assigned to each pixel by solving simultaneous equations by filtered back projection. The x-ray linear attenuation coefficient (μ) is directly related to the CT number of the tissue in that voxel, and the standard scale of CT numbers involves the Hounsfield scale of Hounsfield units (HU) that are distinct from heat units. The Hounsfield scale shows that dense bone measures at 1000 HU, whereas water measures at 0 HU and air measures at −1000 HU. A single Hounsfield unit (HU) equals 0.1% of the difference between the μ of tissue and the μ of water. Although the Hounsfield scale ranges from −1000 to +1000, some imagers use a CT number scale of −2000 to +6000.

Affects on image: The brightness of the pixel is proportional to the Hounsfield Unit (HU): a pixel with a high HU is bright, whereas a pixel with a low HU is dark. The video monitor associated with the CT can display approximately 256 different shades of gray, although the naked eye can detect only approximately 20 of those shades. The range of CT numbers displayed is called the window width (WW); the central value is called the window level (WL). Any reduction of the WW increases the contrast. The CT number at the center of the displayed gray scale is the WL. The WW and the WL allow practitioners to visualize the entire CT or HU number scale.

Window width and window level

A wide window width (WW) is most often used by practitioners to complete bone imaging, whereas a narrow WW is used to complete soft-tissue imaging. Window size or windowing refers to the manipulations of the window level (WL) and WW that are necessary for optimizing the image contrast. Wide WW produces a gray image that has a long gray scale and low contrast, whereas a narrow WW produces a higher-contrast black-and-white image with a short gray scale and high contrast. The CT image produced is optimized for the tissue that has the same CT number as the WL. The Hounsfield Scale for bones ranges from +1000 HU to +300 HU, whereas that for soft tissue ranges from +200 HU to −100 HU and that for lung tissues ranges from −300 HU to −800 HU.

Typical WW and WL viewing: The posterior fossa of the brain has 100 WW and 40 WL, whereas the brain itself has 80 WW and 40 WL. Soft tissue in the chest has 400 WW and 40 WL, whereas the lung has 1500 WW and −400 WL. The abdomen is similar to the soft tissue of the chest, at 400 WW and 50 WL. Soft tissue of the C-spine has 500 WW and 60 WL, whereas the bone has 1600 WW and 300 WL. Soft tissue of the T-spine also has 500 WW and 60 WL, with the bone at 1600 WW and 300 WL. Soft tissue of the orbit has 400 WW and 30 WL, whereas the brain has 100 WW and 40 WL and the bone has 3000 WW and 500 WL. Temporal bone has 3000 WW and 500 WL, whereas the spine has 1600 WW and 300 WL.

Cine

Practitioners using cine CT to examine the mediastinum in pediatric patients can image neoplastic, inflammatory, and vascular lesions in a view that is clearer than that of traditional CT. With a scan time of less than 50 ms, cine CT produces images that provide an excellent depiction of the heart and the airway. Cine CT enables practitioners to minimize motion artifact, to follow through with the examinations that are to be completed with little or no sedation, and to allow for optimal opacification of all vascular structures with as little as 0.5 mL of intravenously administered contrast per kilogram of body weight. The scanning time required for obtaining 20 image sections is approximately 10 s. The dose of radiation required for cine CT is lower than that required for comparable CT or radiographic studies.

Region of interest

Region of interest (ROI) is a specific studied area of anatomy as viewed on a reconstructed digital CT image that could be drawn or selected by the operator in a circular, square, elliptical, rectangular, or custom-drawn fashion for purposes of the study. Practitioners must define the ROI in the initial stages of the study so that further definitions relating to the number of image displays and measurement functions can also be delineated. If the ROI changes or is modified, then the other corresponding steps must also be likewise modified.

Dose reduction: Continuous studies and applications of CT scanning have allowed practitioners to observe dramatically improved CT image quality. By reducing the imaged volume to a specific region of interest (ROI), practitioners can reduce the integral dose, although this reduction may result in additional artifacts. Several techniques have been used to recover accurate reconstructions with a minimal amount of artifact when the ROI data are obtained. Such techniques include providing no dose to the area outside the ROI through collimation, lowering the dose for the area outside the ROI with a filter in the beam, or lowering the dose outside the ROI with a separate acquisition with lower technique factors. The data inside and outside the ROI can be appropriately normalized and combined so as to provide practitioners with an accurate reconstruction in the ROI. Finally, the differences between ROI and FFOV reconstructions could reach 1% to 2% for dose reduction.

Biopsy, WW, and WL: CT-guided biopsy can be used to localize lesions by using the ROI feature for clarification. Practitioners can follow radiopaque markers to help guide the needle to the area of interest during the biopsy in conjunction with the spiral CT, which permits the practitioner to image the entire liver and pancreas at a certain time phase, including arterial, portal, or venous. Bone imaging requires a wide WW (e.g., 500 to 1000) and low WL (e.g., 40 to 60), whereas lung imaging requires a wide WW (e.g., 700 to 900) and high WL (e.g., 800). Abdominal and pelvic imaging, on the other hand, requires a narrow WW (e.g., 200 to 400) and low WL (e.g., 40 to 60), although CT fluoroscopy is most useful for angiointervention in the abdomen and chest, producing 8 images per second for near real-time imaging.

Filtration

Filtration is the removal of low-energy x-rays from the useful beam with a metal such as aluminum. This removal results in an increase in beam quality and a reduction in patient dose. The filter itself is an added material designed to increase the effective x-ray energy through the absorption of low-energy x-rays. CT x-ray beams are filtered to make the beams more uniform at the detector array and to harden their projection. The filtration produces higher energy, a more homogenous x-ray beam, and less beam-hardening artifact. The x-ray beam filter is shaped to produce an intensity that is more uniform at the detector array, although some facilities often incorporate a bow tie filter to even the intensity at the detector array.

Post-processing

Post-processing in CT includes an image pan and zoom; distance and area analysis; histogram analysis; annotation; quantitative CT; multi-image display; windowing; contrast control and reversal; image rotation; and the collage and coronal, sagittal, and oblique reconstruction, enhancement, and smoothing. The completion of post-processing will not yield any additional information for the image but will provide the practitioner with a different presentation of the same or less information. Many widely applied multiplanar reconstruction (MPR) algorithms produce maximum intensity projection (MIP) and shaded-surface display (SSD). Multiplanar reconstruction results in coronal and sagittal images from stacked transverse images, whereas quantitative CT (QCT) relates vertebral bone CT numbers with standard phantoms imaged simultaneously to assay bone mineralization.

Features of post-processing

The post-processing function associated with CT involves different features for accurate completion and review. Such features include the change contrast scale, which could be different for each CT scan, considering the area being scanned, the density of the material there, and the contrast material used, if any. The ROI for the QCT would also affect post-processing, because the comparison of the CT numbers will differ in separate regions. The linear and volume measurement will also be individualized for each CT scan, as will the surface and volume rendering. Finally, CT angiography will address multiplanar imaging, the analysis of the vessel wall and lumen, and the injection of contrast material, but it must also have a separate area for post-processing.

3-D rendering

Maximum intensity projection: Multiple maximum intensity projection (MIP) images can be reconstructed at different angles while being viewed in rotation so that the practitioner can separate the superimposed vessels inherent in the image. Although first employed in MRI technology, the MIP function is the basis of computed tomography angiography (CTA). The proper image plane can be created by the practitioner, who must have a good foundation in the anatomical structuring of the body, specifically the vascular anatomy. MIP focus is directed at select voxels that are ranged along a row or column in a volume of interest (VOI) with the highest CT number or a certain range of CT numbers in the display. Bones frequently have higher CT numbers than contrast-filled vessels and so must be excluded in the software analysis.

The multiple overlapping reconstruction of the MIP reduces the beading artifact that occasionally appears in the MIP because the voxel with the highest CT number is displayed along any row column. The voxels that are enhanced with contrast material are displayed in order first before soft-tissue voxels out of preference. Although MIP images do not provide the practitioner with any degree of depth, those images are susceptible to volume and so are classified as volume-rendered images. The shaded surfaces of the SSD are classified as surface-rendered images, and the width of the ROI should be as small as possible in MIP so as to reduce any background noise that might occur in the presence of contrast-filled vessels.

Spiral CT: Already considered important in CT examinations, post-processing of spiral CT information should become a requirement for that part of radiological practice. The views offered from film to monitor displays show the interactive post-processing tools that are used to support the evaluation of CT studies and that are in many cases improving the diagnostic accuracy of the information. Axial images and multiplanar reformats (MPR) may require track-ball–controlled browsing through the volume of data, and these tools can become integral to most of the CT evaluations that are performed. MPR and three-dimensional displays already act as important adjuncts for most orthopaedic and trauma applications. Three-dimensional surface displays and MIPs are routine display modalities in CTA. The new volume-rendering techniques (VRT) used with interactive parameter changes are making three-dimensional imaging of soft tissues more feasible.

Spiral CT datasets have high z-axis resolution, as shown by subsecond scanning, thin collimation, and overlapping image reconstruction, as well as an optimized application of the contrast material. The ability to communicate post-processing information with the referring physician by using three-dimensional representations has become increasingly important in the practitioner's ability to monitor treatment planning and control. The importance of the services available through post-processing has increased for successful radiological practices. More facilities have subscribed to the notion that practitioners should perform post-processing at their own initiative until the facility institutes such capabilities. Post-processing can assist practitioners who see treatment simulation, virtual surgical instruments, and tissue motion models as being in the early stages of development.

The z-axis resolution is better with 180° interpolation than with 360° interpolation, although the 180° interpolation results in a thinner slice than the 360° interpolation. Occasionally practitioners will be required to extrapolate values, which means that they must compute an unknown value by using the known values of one side of the equation. Noisier images are produced with the 180° interpolation, although the 180° interpolation of spiral CT has about 20% more noise than conventional CT. Conversely, the 360° interpolation has 20% less noise than conventional CT. Z-axis resolution is better in 180° interpolation than on reformatted longitudinal images, and the 180° interpolation allows the scanning to be completed at a higher pitch. The 360° interpolation broadens the sensitivity profile and produces less noise than the 180° interpolation, although both use linear and higher-order reconstruction algorithms.

Data management

Hard copy and soft copy

Hard-copy information refers to printed CT images or reproduced paper forms. Soft-copy information refers to stored CT images displayed on either a cathode ray tube (CRT) or a flat panel display or stored on either magnetic or optical disks. Practitioners have discovered that if all information is to be attached to the medical record, some of that information must be printed out in hard copy and physically attached to a file. The amount of memory required for producing and viewing CT images dissuades many practitioners from maintaining a soft-copy file of the pertinent information. However, hard-copy forms or test results may be misfiled, and the sensitive information they contain may be revealed to an unapproved party. Many facilities require that the medical files be stored as soft copy and that hard-copy folders be prepared for transference and review by approved parties.

Storage and transfer

As with all procedures in the healthcare facility, the transference of data must conform to the approved protocol because of the sensitive nature of the information and the privacy rights of the patients. DICOM data can be stored on CD, DVD, or Optical Disk on Unix, Mac, Linux, and Windows machines. Some facilities will also allow Pioneer 702 or 502 LaserMemory, Sony, Maxoptix, and Verbatim optical disks with a format size of 650 MB to 9.1 GB. For optical disk data storage, jpeg images should not be included with e-film; DICOM images should be selected while the CD is being made. With GE CT or high-speed advantage helical CT, practitioners should save images by using standard archives; with Imatron, the images should be saved as uncompressed when transferred to CD or optical disk.

With Picker CT, practitioners should save images in uncompressed format archives with 1 patient data per disk and a standard backup tape, which should be an 8-mm data cartridge similar to a Sony QG-112M. With Phillips CT, practitioners should use the Archive Images from the Easy Vision Workstation to save images onto an optical disk in the Easy Vision uncompressed format. With the comparable Phillips TomoVision, however, practitioners should save the images in HDL format. With Shimadzu, practitioners should save images by using the standard optical disk archives. Practitioners with Siemens CT should use the uncompressed archive option for optical disk storage. With Toshiba CT, practitioners should save images by using the standard optical disk archives.

Electronic transmission

A thinner collimation is generally preferred when the practitioner must cover a particular length of patient anatomy in the test and scanning. The combination of the thinner collimation and higher pitch produces better spatial resolution. When the pitch exceeds the 2-to-1 ratio, it is not clinically useful because of broadened sensitivity profile and reduced z-axis resolution. The higher pitch used in spiral CT will result in a thinner slice thickness and will subsequently produce less partial-volume artifact. When the pitch is greater than 1 in spiral CT, the sensitivity profile is wider than that of conventional CT. With higher pitch, practitioners can attain a wider sensitivity profile, although the sensitivity of spiral CT is described by the full width at tenth maximum (FWTM) instead of the conventional full width at half maximum (FWHM).

Image Quality

Image quality is defined by the spatial resolution, contrast resolution, image noise, linearity, and uniformity of the CT images. Although the specification of the image quality is very subjective, terms such as detail, recorded detail, sharpness, and blur are used to objectively describe the images obtained by CT scanning. This quality cannot be represented by a single number because several facets contribute to the quality of the image; therefore, several numbers are used to represent the quality of the image. Although the quality cannot be delineated by a single number, the facets of image quality (i.e., spatial resolution, contrast resolution, image noise, linearity, and uniformity) can be described numerically and compiled for determining the quality of the final image.

Spatial resolution

Spatial resolution is the ability to faithfully reproduce small objects that have the high subject contrast of the original object being imaged. The interface represented by bone and soft tissue shows a very high subject contrast, whereas the interface represented by liver and spleen shows a very low subject contrast. A sharp bone and soft tissue interface is described as having a high spatial frequency interface, although high spatial frequency objects are more difficult to image than low spatial frequency objects. Spatial resolution itself is often referred to as the level of blurring that is seen in the image so that small, high-contrast objects can be more difficult to image than large, low-contrast objects.

Affecting spatial resolution

A larger pixel size will result in a poorer spatial resolution, and the lower subject contrast will also result in poorer spatial resolution. A larger detector size can also result in poorer spatial resolution. Smaller x-ray tube focal spots improve spatial resolution due to the sharper image projection and not the geometry of the shadow. One method for evaluating spatial resolution includes point response function (PRF), though practitioners may also consider edge response function (ERF) or line spread function (LSF). As a mathematical manipulation, the Fourier transform (FT) converts an intensity versus distance relationship into an intensity versus 1/distance spatial frequency relationship. In this way, the FT of a PRF and an ERF will result in a modulation transfer function (MTF), while the FT of an LSF will also result in an MTF.

Improving spatial resolution

Spatial resolution can be aptly described as limiting the spatial frequency (lp/cm). The MTF can be useful for evaluating the components of a system or for comparing similar systems. Thinner-section imaging and narrow predetector collimation will improve spatial resolution, as will a longer source-to-isocenter distance. Practitioners can also improve spatial resolution by using an edge enhancement reconstruction algorithm, such as a convolution, or by increasing the number of projection profiles that are acquired per scan. Small FOV or larger matrix can also improve the spatial resolution. At high spatial frequencies the MTF is classified as a measure of the spatial resolution and acts as the principal means of expressing the CT spatial resolution.

MTF and spatial frequency

Spatial frequency is composed of units of line pairs/mm (lp/mm) so that 1 line and a line-sized interspace complete 1 line-pair (lp). Small objects are represented by high spatial frequencies, whereas large objects are represented by low spatial frequencies. When an MTF reaches the value of 1.0, the practitioner has an absolutely perfect image. As the MTF value decreases, the image blur increases, and the quality of the image is reduced. The limiting resolution is the spatial frequency observed at 0.1 MTF, and the total MTF of an imager is determined by the product of the component MTFs. CT imagers can produce almost 10 lp/cm (1 lp/mm) in a normal mode and can produce almost 20 lp/cm (2 lp/mm) in a high-resolution mode. The z-axis resolution of the MTF is better with spiral CT than with conventional CT.

Influences on spatial resolution

Practitioners can determine the quality of the spatial resolution by using objects that have a large signal-to-noise ratio and measuring the system's ability to resolve the high-contrast objects of consistently smaller sizes or increasing spatial frequencies. High spatial resolution is influenced by the system's geometric resolution limits, such as the focal spot size, detector width, and ray sampling; pixel size; and properties of the convolution kernel and mathematical reconstruction filter. Practitioners have noted that using reconstruction filters that preserve or enhance the higher spatial frequencies or smaller objects often results in higher levels of noise in the image. This difference could be acceptable when imaging objects with a high signal-to-noise ratio, but it can compromise the quality of the image for other objects.

Contrast resolution

Improving contrast resolution

CT imaging proffers superior contrast resolution because of the narrow x-ray beam collimation, which allows for excellent scatter radiation rejection. Practitioners can improve contrast resolution with a larger pixel size, high mAs, thick image slices, and a low-pass filter. A larger dynamic range, such as 2^{10} (1024) rather than 2^9 (512), produces less contrast in the image. MTF is a measure of the lower spatial frequencies. Practitioners use contrast resolution to image adjacent tissues that are similar in mass density and effective atomic number, although they can improve that contrast resolution by using a higher mA or thicker image slices. Contrast resolution is better when patients are smaller and when low-noise imagers are used. A larger FOV, a smaller matrix size, and the addition of a smoothing reconstruction filter can combine to improve contrast resolution.

Low-contrast resolution

Practitioners can produce low-contrast resolution by providing a very small difference, such as a 4- to 10-HU distinction, between the object and the background. The signal, or the difference between the object and the background, is so small that the noise becomes an important factor in the test, which measures the system's ability to resolve low-contrast objects of consistently smaller sizes or increasing spatial frequencies. The most widely accepted method of resolving the recognition of low-contrast objects involves having an observer subjectively determine the contrast of the smaller objects as being distinct, even though several purely quantitative methods have been proposed and discussed in related literature.

Noise

The quality of a CT image depends several interlinked factors. Contrast resolution and noise detract from the quality of the image and are interconnected in the modifications of the CT scan. Low-contrast resolution and noise interfere with each other but can also be influenced by such outside factors as window width and window level settings, the film or monitor calibration curve, the specificity of the printed image, the clarity and color-contrast capability of the computer monitor, the viewing conditions, the patient, the practitioner, and other medical personnel who are observing. Noise that is created by different mAs levels (e.g., 240 mAs and 80 mAs) can also affect the low-contrast resolution, and this effect could affect the quality of the image.

Image noise

In its most basic form, image noise is classified in CT scanning as the standard deviation of voxel values in a homogenous phantom, such as water or another simple liquid. Some practitioners have broadened this definition to include such additional factors as the contrast scale of the scanner or the viewing capabilities of the medical equipment at the healthcare facility. Image noise is greatly influenced by factors such as kVp, mA, collimation and reconstructed slice thickness, exposure time, helical interpolation algorithm, reconstruction algorithm or filter, helical pitch or table speed, focal spot to isocenter distance, detector deficiency. Practitioners expect a reduction of mAs to increase the measured standard deviation in noise, although some practitioners are hesitant to increase mAs for the sake of a cleaner image at the expense of the patient.

Increasing or decreasing noise

Image noise limits contrast resolution, but scatter radiation also results in image noise on CT scans. Research has shown that practitioners who increase the slice thickness of the CT scan notice less noise in the images, and this increase in slice thickness will usually result in a decrease in patient dose. Increasing pixel size or patient dose will also reduce the amount of noise that practitioners must interpret on CT scans. High-noise images often appear grainy, blotchy, or spotty, whereas low-noise images appear less animated and often smooth. The quality of the image can be adjusted by improving contrast resolution and, subsequently, reducing CT noise; conversely, any reduction in CT noise will improve contrast resolution. A 360° interpolation will reduce image noise, and the low-pass convolution filter can accommodate increased image noise at low mAs levels.

Quality assurance procedures

All CT components should be maintained and monitored so that accurate testing results can be ensured. CT noise can be evaluated by scanning a water bath that has a standard deviation not to exceed ±10. The CT number of water should be calculated at 0, and the spatial resolution should equal at least the manufacturer's specifications. Practitioners who scan a water phantom should select region of interest (ROI) that is large enough to allow a CT number of ±3. Practitioners who scan an empty gantry aperture should also select an ROI that is large enough to allow the CT number for air to be–1000 ± 5. Practitioners can evaluate spatial resolution by scanning any number of phantom-hole patterns or line-pair patterns. Contrast resolution can be evaluated with thick or thin phantoms with various hole sizes filled with water or with various hole sizes of differing depths for partial-volume effects.

Equipment specifications

Most CT imagers can attain images at 0.5 mm (10 lp/cm), although some can attain an image at 0.2 mm (20 lp/cm) in a high-resolution mode. With these types of results, the contrast resolution should be at least 5 mm at 5% contrast. The distance measurement accuracy of the CT is measured and determined by the American Association of Physicists in Medicine (AAPM) during their evaluation with a test object that contains pins separated by 10-mm intervals. The AAPM evaluates the degree of distortion of the video monitor used by pressing a clear plastic ruler against the screen image of the 10-mm pin test object so that they can ensure the 5% accuracy. Any electronic distance calipers must be accurate to within ±5%.

The scan plane localization of the CT being studied should be accurate to within 1 mm, although the scan plane is usually a laser light localizer. Research and development has also made available many test devices for scan plane localization. Practitioners or other medical personnel can check the indexing for the patient couch by placing distinct marks or film that has been wrapped in cardboard on the couch and rail. The limit of error for this type of monitoring is 1%. The slice width of the CT imager can usually be evaluated with a ramp test object, and it should be within 50% for nominal widths of 5 mm or higher with no less than 100% for thinner slices.

Phantoms

Practitioners can use high-precision, commercially available phantoms when performing quality assurance procedures for such specialized evaluations as stereotactic radiosurgery treatments. Such quantitative evaluations for system uncertainties such as imaging, treatment delivery systems, and planning can provide practitioners with quality assurance tests that can show how well-defined the targets are and can suggest the direction of further research. Most imaging modalities can identify targets of superior definition within ±1 mm when targets are reproduced within 2 cm^3 in CT and MRI and delivered within 2% of the prescribed dose and within 2-mm accuracy. With additional research, practitioners can gauge the tolerance and appropriate planning system for establishing baseline comparisons and frequency of testing.

Radiation dose

Practitioners use phantoms to determine an effective patient dose and to compare such parameters as exposure time, kVp, mA, x-ray beam collimation, pitch or table speed, the specifics of the scanner being used, dose reduction options such as techniques for modulating tube current, the distance from the focal point to the isocenter, and indirect effects of algorithm and collimation. Addressing these individual parameters can help practitioners reduce noise levels and patient dose and can improve the quality of the image. The quality of the CT image can be dramatically improved by reducing the tube current or mA, increasing the table increment on the axial or the pitch, developing mA settings that are more reflective of the patient's weight or diameter and the particular body region being scanned, reducing the number of multiple scans by including contrast materials, and eliminating inappropriate referrals for CT.

Tradeoffs between image quality and radiation dose

A reduction in patient dose is often preferable for the condition of the patient, although such a reduction may compromise the quality of the image. Practitioners must determine at what point the health of the patient should be considered in light of improving the image by making changes to the parameters of the test or to the patient's exposure and limit. Reductions in mAs will result in reduced radiation dose proportionate to the mAs but will also increase image noise. Increasing the speed or pitch of the table speed will result in reduced radiation dose proportionate to the increase in pitch but may increase the slice sensitivity profile to create larger effective slice thickness and reduced z-axis resolution. Because some machines will automatically increase mA with any increase in pitch, changing pitch is not always considered a viable alternative.

When practitioners reduce kVp, they may witness a reduction in radiation dose that may not be linear with kVp. Alternatively, they may see an increased signal contrast for certain tissues and for iodine with its high z-axis resolution, as a result of an increase in photoelectric response. Reductions in kVp may also significantly increase the beam-hardening artifact if the beam energy drops to 80 kVp. When thinner slices or high spatial frequency filters are used while other factors remain constant, noise increases; this noise may cause the practitioner to increase mAs, which will increase the radiation dose. Some tests will have higher signal-to-noise ratios, such as those used to detect a solid nodule in the lung or a calcium deposit in a coronary artery. Other tests will produce lower signal-to-noise ratios, such as scans for diffuse lung disease and abdominal scans.

Linearity

The CT imager reflects perfect linearity with CT numbers for air at –1000, for water at 0, and for bone at 1000. The CT number for any given tissue is determined by the x-ray linear attenuation coefficient (μ). A plot of CT numbers contrasted with μ should result in a straight line that intersects water at 0. QCT depends heavily on solid linearity, because the level of linearity determines the ability of the CT imager to correctly categorize the correct Hounsfield unit (HU) to any particular tissue. Medical facilities can monitor the quality of the linearity in CT imagers by imaging the 5-pin insert of the American Association of Physicists in Medicine (AAPM) and using that information to plot the HU against the linear attenuation coefficient.

Uniformity

To be considered uniform, an object must image with an equal value for each pixel on the basis of the groups of substances in the physical make-up of the object. Practitioners may observe either cupping, which is a reduction in the CT number toward the middle of the uniform test object, or peaking, which is an increase in the CT number toward the middle of the uniform test object. Both cupping and peaking are signs of poor image uniformity. QCT depends on image uniformity.

Contrast-detail

Contrast-detail has a noise-limited curve in the low-contrast region, because that curve is determined by the MTF of the imager when high-contrast regions are evaluated. The associated plots are useful for evaluating contrast resolution and spatial resolution and for comparing various scanning protocols.

Artifact Recognition and Reduction

Image artifacts

Any motion by the patient, whether that motion is voluntary or involuntary, results in a motion artifact, a pattern appearing on an image that does not accurately represent the anatomy and does not exist in real life. Artifacts may also be caused by equipment characteristics or operator error, although artifacts may also be classified as unintended optical density appearing on any radiograph or associated film-type image. Appearing as streaks or step-like patterns at high-contrast edges, artifacts result from incomplete projection profiles in the x-ray absorption. Metal in certain tissues can image as streaks or star-shaped artifacts. Respiratory motion artifacts may mimic vascular stenosis or aneurysm on CTA images and could thus be misinterpreted as a serious condition rather than being recognized as an artifact.

Beam hardening

The x-ray beam penetrates cranial bone and is selectively hardened and filtered. This process may produce an image with a false low linear attenuation coefficient and a false low CT number. The beam-hardening artifact may appear on the screen as a dark ring inside the cranial bone with cupping at the center of the image. If any calcification or other object also exists in the area but is not fully inside the slice thickness, the image will indicate a false CT number for that object. The artifact itself results from lower-energy photons that are preferentially absorbed by the tissue surrounding the target to leave higher-energy photons to collide with the detector array.

Partial-volume artifacts

Although practitioners can reduce the appearance of partial volume artifacts by overlapping scans, this method requires increasing the patient dose to achieve clearer and more accurate images. Thinner slice thicknesses can also be used to reduce the appearance of partial-volume artifacts, although this method will cause higher noise levels in the image and will require the patient to absorb a higher dose of radiation. Spiral CT can produce images with fewer partial-volume artifacts simply by moving the plane of reconstruction, and the multiple reconstruction of the spiral CT following the z-axis will also reduce partial-volume artifacts. Practitioners can reduce the appearance of partial-volume artifacts by combining several thin-slice reconstructed images.

Motion artifacts

Practitioners who observe motion artifacts are usually not familiar with methods of solving for inconsistencies in attenuation during the reconstruction. These methods rely on the computer to place attenuation values into a matrix, which is a grid showing columns and rows of small sections (pixels). An effective attenuation value can be placed at the proper address if the patient moves during the CT; this means that the computer can manipulate only the data that have been deemed necessary for correct evaluation. Practitioners can prevent motion artifacts by establishing quicker scan times, such as 50 ms, by using high-speed scanners or ECG gating to synchronize the data with the patient's heartbeat; gating techniques, such as single-breathhold ECG gating; and signal processing, which comprises different approaches for categorizing organ motion.

Metal artifacts

Caused by high-density objects, usually those made of metal, metal artifacts appear on CT images as streaks. They can result from scanning objects such as dental fillings, surgical clips, or metal prosthetic devices. The resultant streaks occur because the imaged objects exceed the maximum attenuation value that the CT imager can produce. Older CT scans use 1000 as the maximum attenuation number because that is the CT number of cortical bone, the densest natural structure in the human body. Because metal objects are generally denser than cortical bone, practitioners must expand the CT number scales to avoid metal artifacts. Alternatively, they can reduce the appearance of metal artifacts by using postreconstruction algorithms to remove metal objects from the image and then using projection-completion methods to find the data missing because of removal of the metal object.

Edge gradient

An edge gradient effect occurs during CT scanning when long, sharp edges of high contrast are encountered. The effect is nonlinear and is caused by the interaction of the width of the scanning beam and the x-ray attenuation. The most common effect on the image is the appearance of lucent streaks from single straight edges, although it is also possible to see dense streaks arising from pairs of edges. Increasing the sample density can help practitioners correcting these edge gradient errors. Appropriate correction algorithms have been shown to work well with simulated CT phantom scans by providing approximately 4 samples per beam width. The slice thickness or sensitivity profile is controlled by the postpatient collimator.

Equipment induced artifacts

Third-generation CT imagers may produce ring artifacts caused by malfunction of the detector. Pulsation artifacts occur during CTA and may mimic vascular stenosis. Practitioners can reduce the occurrence of pulsation artifacts by incorporating the 360° interpolation in lieu of the 180° interpolation. Stair-step artifacts occur most commonly during spiral CT examinations, and the artifacts themselves are most obvious on the inclined vessels during spiral CTA. The height of the stair-step artifact is often proportionate to the couch increment but is independent of the reconstruction interval or collimation. Practitioners must become familiar with the appearance of the images from the various CT tests and with the artifacts that can occur during imaging so that they can make a correct diagnosis on the basis of image artifacts.

Important Terms

Assay is the physical act of examining and determining the characteristics, such as weight, quality, or measure, of a particular object. An analysis of an ore or medication, for instance, is also classified as an assay, which serves to verify the presence, absence, or quantity present in one or more mechanisms of the object under study.

X-ray is a type of ionizing electromagnetic radiation with high energy that has a wavelength much shorter than the wavelengths of visible light.

Carcinogenic is a term describing any outside agent or substance that can produce or incite the growth of cancerous cells in a living body.

Computed tomography (CT) creates a transverse, or across-the-body, tomographic section that is produced by incorporating a rotating fan beam, computed reconstruction, and a detector array. A CT scan can decrease the need for invasive, risky procedures.

Gantry is the framework that holds the x-ray tube and the radiation detection system. It can also include the portion of the CT or magnetic resonance imager that is used to accommodate patients, sources, and detector assemblies.

Fan beam is an x-ray beam pattern that is commonly used in CT. Fan beams are projected as slits.

Detector is a device that measures the intensity of x-ray beams and maintains sensitivity to the x-rays projected.

Detector array is a group of detectors and the interspace materials that are used to separate them. The image receptor in CT is a detector array.

Diaphragm is a device used to restrict the projected x-ray beam to a fixed size as determined by the practitioner and the area of the patient being studied.

Detector efficiency is the ability of the detector to capture the transmitted x-ray beams and to transfer those beams into electronic signals that can be mapped out as a digital image.

Geometric efficiency is determined by the fraction of the actual detector area that intercepts the x-ray beam. The portion of area not included is called the interspace.

Quantum detection efficiency (QDE) is determined by the relative number of x-ray beams that interact with the detector. Higher numbers can provide clearer images, but they also increase the likelihood that patients will respond negatively to the level of radiation.

Quantum theory is the physics of electromagnetic radiation and the branch of science that uses those particles of matter that are smaller than atoms.

Kerma (k) is the energy that is absorbed per unit mass from an initial kinetic energy released in matter or the total electrons that have been liberated by x-rays or gamma rays. Expressed in gray (Gy), kerma can be shown as 1 Gy = 1 J/kg; air kerma is expressed as Gy_a, and tissue dose is expressed as Gy_1.

Joule (J) is a unit of energy in which the work completed is represented as a force of 1 N acting on an object with an area of 1 m and is equivalent to 1 HU.

Kiloelectron volt (keV) is a measure of energy that is equivalent to 1000 eV.

Kilovolt is a measure of high voltage that is produced by the x-ray generator or the qualitative measure of the x-ray beam.

Milliampere seconds (mAs) are the product of exposure time and the x-ray tube currently best exemplified by the total number of electrons used to produce the x-ray beam in the CT.

Milliampere (mA) is the measure of the x-ray tube current that is used during the production of x-rays. Milliampere is also the quantitative measure of the x-ray beam when combined with the imaging time.

Mass is the quantity of matter measured in kilograms.

Matter is any object that has a form or shape and occupies space.

Power is the time-rate at which work is completed, as well as the rate of change in the amount of energy over time. Power is expressed in watts (W) where 1 W = 1 J/s.

Absorption is the transfer of energy from radiation to objects of matter, including the removal of x-rays from a beam through the photoelectric effect.

Absorber is any material that is characterized by its ability to absorb or reduce the intensity of the exposed radiation.

Added filtration is aluminum or comparable metal of the appropriate thickness to be positioned near an x-ray tube and maintain its chemical components in the primary beam.

Aperture is a circular opening in the gantry of the CT or magnetic resonance imager whereby a patient may enter the machine and be tested. Aperture can also refer to a fixed collimation of a diagnostic x-ray tube or the variable opening in front of the lens of a photo- or cinespot camera.

Anode is the positive side of the x-ray tube that also contains the target.

Cathode is the negative side of the x-ray tube that contains both the focusing cup and the filament.

Area beam is the x-ray beam pattern used in conventional radiography and fluoroscopy; it is commonly shaped like a square or a rectangle.

Array processor is the portion of the computer that will accept the signal data and perform the mathematical calculations necessary for reconstructing a digital image.

Central processing unit (CPU) is the main part of the computer that accepts information from the DAS and reconfigures that information to form an accurate and detailed image for medical diagnostics and treatment.

Attenuation is the reduction in the intensity of radiation when it passes through matter, whereupon that radiation is absorbed and scattered.

Attenuator is the material or device used to reduce the intensity of x-ray or ultrasound.

Attenuation profile is the result of the CT process that defines the attenuation properties of individual ray sums as they relate to the position of the ray.

Attenuation coefficient is the numerical expression of a decrease in intensity that includes a penetration into matter. Also defined by the process of energy absorption, the attenuation coefficient describes the percent of radiation that remains after the x-rays pass through an object. It is expressed as an inverse length of m^{-1} or cm^{-1}.

Radiation quality is the relative penetrability of any x-ray beam as it travels through matter. It is determined by the average amount of energy, usually measured in HVL or kVp.

Radiation quantity is the intensity of the radiation or x-ray beams being aimed at any one patient and, if possible, deflected off any particular surface. Radiation quantity is usually measured in mR or by Gy_a air kerma.

Radiation standards are the recommendations, regulations, and rules for any healthcare facility regarding the permitted concentrations, transportation, safe handling techniques, and control of the radioactive material being studied and possibly transported between facilities.

Radiation safety officer (RSO) is a qualified person who has been designated by an institution to verify that the facility and medical personnel are following the accepted guidelines for radiation protection.

Protocol is the process that is used to perform any quality-control measurement or associated procedure. Distinct protocols are relative to various procedures, and all practitioners should be cognizant of this differentiation when completing the specific procedure on a patient.

Quality assurance (QA) involves all of the systematic and planned actions that are needed for providing adequate confidence that a system, facility, or administrative component will perform satisfactory and safe services for patients. Scheduling, preparation, and promptness in both examination and treatment are important in QA, as are the reporting of results and quality control.

Quality control involves all of the actions that are necessary for controlling and verifying the performance of the equipment.

Image reconstruction is the use of raw data to create a CT image.

Edge gradient effect is the straight-line artifacts that can radiate or extend from a high-contrast area in CT. Edge gradient effect is most commonly seen in images of bone and soft tissue.

Display field of view (also called target view and zoon) is a measure of how much raw data is used to display a CT image.

Scanned field of view (also called calibration field) is the area within the gantry at which the raw data of the CT image are obtained.

View is the complete set of ray sums that, when combined, produce a single CT image.

Ray sum is the measurement of how much the x-ray beam has been attenuated as determined by the detector.

Volume averaging is the process used to find a voxel that contains different tissue; the CT numbers of those tissues are averaged to produce a specific CT number that is unrelated to either component.

Partial volume effect is the distortion of signal intensity from an object that partially extends into the adjacent slice thickness. Also known as volume averaging, partial volume effect is the process associated with CT by which CT numbers of different tissues can be averaged within a single pixel.

Window level is the location on a CT number scale at which levels of gray are represented by the sample, regulating the optical density of a displayed image. The window level is also the central CT value of the window width.

Window width is either the CT numbers that are assigned to an image or the number of gray levels is that image. The window width regulates the contrast of the displayed images.

Scan parameters are all of the factors that can be manually or deliberately controlled by the practitioner or other medical personnel at the onset and during the testing and that can directly affect the quality of the CT image. Such factors include milliampere, kilovolt peak, slice thickness, scan time, field of view, and algorithm.

Scanner is a device that is used to produce an axial or transverse sectional image. The preferred terminology for the scanner is the imager.

X-ray imager is an x-ray system that is designed for radiography, tomography, or fluoroscopy.

Z-axis is the plane that correlates to the position or slice thickness of a CT slice and is located along the long axis of the CT patient.

Mega is a prefix that multiplies the basic unit by 10^6 or 1 million. Mega is the only prefix in this grouping that multiplies the basic unit.

Micro is a prefix that divides the basic unit by 10^{-6} or 1 million.

Milli is a prefix that divides the basic unit by 10^{-3} or 1 thousand.

Nano is a prefix that divides the basic unit by 10^{-9} or 1 billion.

Pico is a prefix that divides the basic unit by 10^{-12} or 1 trillion.

Rad is the radiation absorbed dose as related to the special unit absorbed dose, so that 1 rad = 100 erg/g = 0.01 Gy.

Rem is the radiation equivalent man as related to the special unit for dose equivalent and effective dose. Rem was replaced by the sievert (SV) in the SI system so that 1 rem = 0.01 Sv.

Use factor (U) is the proportional amount of elapsed time during which the x-ray beam is energized and directed toward a specific barrier.

Vector is any quantity or measurement that has both magnitude and direction.

Work is the product reached by the force exerted on an object and the distance over which that force acts. Work is often expressed in joules (J) so that W = Fd.

Workload (W) is the product reached by the maximum milliamperage (mA) and the total number of x-ray examinations that are performed each week. Workload is expressed in mAmin/wk.

Tungsten is a metal element that is commonly the principal component of the cathode and the anode.

Signal is the information content regarding different degrees of variation contained within the current or voltage as noticed within a receiver.

Signal-to-noise-ratio (SNR) is the sensitivity exhibited by the detector in the process of recognizing a particular signal as it occurs within the context of other types of background noise.

Exposure is the amount of ionization that is produced in the air by x-rays and gamma rays, as well as the amount of ionizing radiation that occurs in living tissue. Exposure is usually expressed in R, C/kg, or air kerma Gy_a.

Ionizing radiation is any form of radiation that is capable of ionization.

Ionization is the removal of an electron from an atom.

Electron is an elementary particle defined by one negative charge. Electrons surround positively charged nuclei and are considered in the classification of the chemical properties associated with each atom.

Electrometer is a device that is commonly used to measure the electric charge of elementary particles; this measurement is useful for determining the chemical properties of the atom.

Ionic and nonionic are the characteristics of contrast materials in relation to their chemical composition. Ionic contrast materials form water in an ion solution, whereas nonionic contrast materials do not dissociate or ionize in water.

Ion is an atom with too many or too few electrons in its association. This electrically charged particle could also contain a free electron, which would make the ion more susceptible to chemical combination with other ions.

Ion pair consists of 2 particles with opposite charges, usually a positively charged atom and an electron.

Isotonic substance has nearly the same number of particles in solution as water.

Photoelectron is an electron that is ejected during the course of the photoelectric effect.

Photoelectric effect is the interaction between an atom and an x-ray in which the x-ray loses its primary identification to the point that an electron is ejected from the inner shell. The term photoelectric effect also refers to the absorption of an x-ray during the process of ionization.

Photon is the smallest quantity of electromagnetic radiation; it can be represented by an x-ray, a gamma ray, or light. Electromagnetic radiation interacts with matter in a manner similar to that of a neutral particle, but it has no mass or electric charge.

Photodiode is a device used to convert light into an electric current in a solid state.

Photoconductor is any type of material that will conduct electrons when that material is illuminated.

Particulate radiation consists of alpha particles, electrons, neutrons, and protons that are distinctly separate from x-rays and gamma rays.

Filament is that portion of the cathode that emits the electrons that result in the x-ray tube current.

Space charge is the cloud of electrons that forms near the filament.

Target is the region of the anode that is struck by the electrons emitted by the filament. This term is also used to describe the source of x-radiation.

Thermionic emission is the emission of electrons from the surface of a heated object.

Radiation survey instruments are the area monitoring devices used in medical facilities to detect or measure radiation.

Radiology is a branch of medicine that deals with the diagnostic and therapeutic applications of the radiation used in patient imaging or treatment.

Primary radiation consists of the x-rays that form an image and that emerge from the x-ray tube target that has been confined by collimation to an area of anatomical interest.

Secondary radiation consists of both leakage and scatter radiation.

Leakage radiation consists of the secondary radiation that is emitted through the x-ray tube housing; it does not include the useful beam that is emitted.

Off-focus radiation consists of those x-rays that are emitted from the parts of an anode; it does not include the focal spot.

Remnant radiation refers to all x-rays passing through a patient and interacting with the image receptor.

Protective barrier is an obstruction covered or made with radiation-absorbing material that is used to reduce the exposure of radiation.

Primary protective barrier is the obstruction placed directly in the line of a primary radiation beam.

Secondary protective barrier is the obstruction used to protect against secondary radiation.

Protective apparel consists of specially treated items of clothing, such as aprons and gloves, which provide radiation protection by attenuating x-rays.

Protective housing is a lead-lined metal container that must reduce radiation leakage to 100 mR/m at 1m as it holds the x-ray tube.

Uncontrolled area is a section of the room or department where members of the general public can be located. This area is usually characterized by a lack of protective equipment.

Dose is the amount of energy that has been absorbed by an irradiated object as it relates to the unit mass. Doses are usually expressed in rad or gray (Gy).

Dose equivalent is the quantity of radiation that has been used for radiation protection purposes in expressing dose on a common scale as it relates to all radiations in a particular segment or testing. Dose equivalents are usually expressed in rem or sievert (SV).

Absorbed dose is the energy transferred from the ionizing radiation per unit mass of the irradiated material. Absorbed doses are usually expressed in rad (100 erg/g) or gray (1 J/kg).

Standard is a material or substance whose properties are known accurately enough to allow its incorporation in the evaluation of similar properties of other materials.

Raw data are any measurements that have been obtained from the detector array used in the CT scan.

Scan data are any measurements that have been obtained from the detector array used in the CT scan. The terms raw data and scan data can be used interchangeably.

Scan parameters are the particular factors of the CT scan that are controlled by the operator and that determine the quality of the CT image. Scan parameters usually include milliampere, kilovolt-peak, scan time, algorithm, field of view, and slice thickness.

Spiral CT is the type of scanning CT that continually rotates the x-ray tube with a constant x-ray output and uninterrupted movement of the table. Spiral CT is also referred to as helical, volumetric, or continuous acquisition scanning.

Penetrability is the ability of the x-ray beams to pass through the tissue being imaged. Penetrability can also be used to describe the range in the quality and depth of tissue from the images and the quality of the x-ray.

Reconstruction is the act of creating an image from data, such as the images collected during CT scan.

Reconstruction time is the amount of time after the collection of data during which the computer completes the analysis of the examination information and presents a digital image.

Reformat is the use of the acquired image data to create a particular view but in a different body plane.

Scan is the motion of the detector array and x-ray tube that is necessary for collecting the data used to reconstruct the CT image.

Half scan, also known as partial scan, is the scan that is produced by an x-ray tube arc and normally acquired during a 180° test.

Partial scan is the scan produced by a tube arc of less than 360° and usually acquired from a 180° tube travel in addition to the degree of the arc from the fan angle. The terms partial scan and half scan are used interchangeably.

Overscan is a scan created by a tube travel of 360° in addition to the width of the field of view.

Scout image is to the image used to localize a certain body part.

A **slice** is the thickness of the cross-sectional view of the particular body part that has been scanned for the purpose of regenerating a CT image.

Misregistration is the misalignment of 2 or more images due to the movement of the patient between images.

Slice misregistration is the potential difficulty inherent in the study when a patient breathes inconsistently between acquisition of the various images. This movement could cause some disruption in the images whereby whole sections of anatomy could be missing from the CT study.

Effective slice thickness is the thickness of the CT slice that is actually shown on the CT image; it differs from the size that has been selected by the collimator opening. Effective slice thickness selected in the interpolation of spiral CT could be wider than the selected slice thickness.

Phantom is a device used to simulate most parameters of organs or tissues found in the human body. Phantoms are used to facilitate further study of such issues as pediatric dose equivalent and other sensitive measurements before actual implementation on patients. The use of phantoms is also instrumental in evaluating image performance.

Test object is a passive device similar to a phantom that is also used in measuring and evaluating the performance of CT imagers. Most test objects are created as geometric shapes.

Spectrum is the graphic representation over which the quantity extends in a particular range being studied.

Subtraction is a method used for removing any overlying anatomy in the image so that practitioners can achieve a better view of smaller anatomical structures, such as certain blood vessels in an organ.

Image processor is a component used in a CT system to convert digitized data into shades of gray for ease of interpretation and identification when that data is displayed on a cathode-ray tube monitor.

Inherent filtration is the filtration of useful x-ray beams that is provided by the permanently installed components of the x-ray tube housing assembly in conjunction with the glass window of the x-ray tube.

Resolution is a measure of the quality of the picture taken; it affects the researcher's ability to image objects accurately during CT scanning and to use those images later in further analysis.

Spatial resolution is the ability of the equipment to produce accurate images of anatomical structures or other objects with associated high levels of contrast.

Shadow shield is a shield made of radiopaque material that is held in suspension from a radiographic beam-defining system and is used to cast a shadow visible in the primary that passes directly over the patient.

Radiopaque refers to any tissue or other material that can absorb x-rays but still appear in bright contrast on a radiograph for study and analysis.

Radiolucent refers to any tissue or other material that is known to transmit x-rays while still appearing dark on a radiograph. These tissues or materials are transparent to x-rays.

SOD refers to the source-to-object distance or to the distance between the instrument being used and the organ or tissue being studied.

SSD refers to the source-to-skin distance or the distance between the x-ray tube target and the patient's skin.

Radiation is energy that is emitted from a source and transferred through matter.

Thermal radiation is the transfer of heat by certain emissions of infrared electromagnetic radiation.

Electromagnetic radiation is x-rays, gamma rays, and some nonionizing radiation, including ultraviolet, infrared, and microwave, that can travel at the velocity of light through oscillating electrical and magnetic fields in a vacuum.

Radiation biology is the branch of biological science that studies the effects of ionizing radiation on living systems.

Radiation survey instruments are area monitoring devices that can detect and measure radiation for patients and for practitioners involved in the testing and maintenance areas.

High-contrast resolution is the ability of the scan to image small objects with high subject contrast; it is also referred to as spatial resolution.

Low-contrast resolution is the ability to image objects that have similar subject contrast in the final images.

Image magnification is the post-processing method used to increase proportionally the actual size of the organ or tissue as it appears on the monitor.

Noise is the grainy or uneven appearance of images that results from the use of insufficient numbers of primary x-ray beams. Also classified as uniform signals produced through scattered x-rays, noise can also refer to speckling on images that results when insufficient numbers of x-rays reach the detectors.

CT Practice Test

1. Which of the following questions should be included in the pre-screening for a contrast CT exam on a 35 year old female?
    a. Chance of pregnancy?
    b. Allergies?
    c. Diabetic?
    d. All of the Above

2. State law requires patients to sign consent forms in the following situations:
    a. Prior to any injection of contrast materials
    b. Prior to sedation for surgical procedures
    c. Prior to hospital admission
    d. Signed consent forms are not required by law in all states

3. Thorough patient preparation and education prior to a CT scan will do which of the following?
    a. Reduce repeat radiation exposure
    b. Reduce patient anxiety
    c. Ensure best possible images
    d. All of the above

4. What laboratory test(s) should be performed prior to CT exams that require IV contrast media injections to determine renal function?
    a. Blood Urea Nitrogen (BUN) and Creatinine
    b. Prothrombin Time (PT)
    c. Platelet Count and Complete Blood Count (CBC)
    d. Liver enzymes

5. What is considered a normal range for Blood Urea Nitrogen (BUN)?
    a. 30-55 mg/dl
    b. 0.6-1.7 mg/dl
    c. 5-25 mg/dl
    d. 155-190 mg/dl

6. Which CT Procedure requires Prothrombin Time (PT) and Partial Thromboplastin Time (PTT) laboratory results prior to starting the procedure?
    a. CT abdomen and pelvis with IV contrast
    b. CTA PE chest
    c. CT guided liver biopsy
    d. CT soft tissue neck with IV contrast

7. What method must be utilized for all peripheral venipuncture procedures to reduce the risk of microbial contamination and infection?
    a. Hand washing
    b. Aseptic technique
    c. Proper patient identification
    d. Wearing sterile gloves

8. Peripheral IV access for an optimal CT Angiogram study should meet which criteria:
    a. 20 gauge minimum needle size
    b. Located in the distal extremity
    c. Must have mid-line access
    d. Arterial access must be obtained

9. What are the three phases of IV contrast enhancement?
    a. Velocity, Bolus, Venous
    b. Bolus, Non-Equilibrium, Equilibrium
    c. Equilibrium, Portal Venous, Arterial
    d. Arterial, Venous, Delayed

10. Which factors determine the automatic power injector flow rate during a CT exam?
    a. IV size and location
    b. Type of CT exam
    c. Speed of CT scanner
    d. All of the above

11. What condition is a contraindication to having a patient prep orally with Barium Sulfate?
    a. Diarrhea
    b. Constipation
    c. Tracheoesophageal fistula
    d. Iodine allergy

12. What type of IV contrast agent is rarely used today due to high reaction rates?
    a. Ionic
    b. Non-ionic
    c. Iso-osmolar
    d. Intrathecal

13. What are two negative contrast agents?
    a. Barium sulfate and gastrografin oral contrast
    b. Isomolar and ionic IV contrast
    c. Water and air
    d. Intrathecal and intra-articular contrast

14. What type of IV contrast is the same or less osmolality as blood?
    a. Ionic
    b. Non-ionic
    c. Iso-osmolar
    d. Intrathecal

15. What type of contrast is often used to enhance CT images of the large intestines and the pelvic organs?
    a. Oral barium sulfate
    b. Rectal contrast
    c. Intrathecal contrast
    d. Oral water soluble prep

16. What adrenal pathology may precipitate a hypertensive crisis if IV contrast is utilized?
  a. Multiple myeloma
  b. Diabetes
  c. Pheochromocytoma
  d. Renal insufficiency

17. Why is Multiple Myeloma considered a risk factor and possible contraindication to the injection of IV contrast?
  a. Nephrotoxicity
  b. Anaphylactic reaction
  c. Hypotension
  d. Bronchospasm

18. What adverse reaction category classification do Myocardial Infarction and Respiratory Arrest fall?
  a. Minor
  b. Delayed
  c. Moderate
  d. Severe

19. What contrast media factor(s) is associated with increased instances of adverse reactions to contrast agents?
  a. Higher injection rates
  b. Larger volume of contrast
  c. Higher concentration of iodine
  d. All of the above

20. What effect does warming the contrast agent have on the contrast?
  a. Reduces viscosity
  b. Decreases osmolality
  c. Increases chemo-toxic reactions
  d. Increases viscosity

21. What category of contrast agents is injected into the subarachnoid space during a myelographic study of the spine?
  a. Hyper osmolar
  b. Intra-articular
  c. Intrathecal
  d. Intravenous ionic

22. Diabetic patients should refrain from taking what medication post IV contrast injection and resume only after renal function has been determined to be normal?
  a. Beta blockers
  b. Insulin
  c. Coumadin
  d. Metformin

23. What imaging parameter is defined as the extent to which the x-ray helix is stretched during a helical scan, determines volume covered, and affects radiation exposure and image quality?

   a. Pitch
   b. Table increment
   c. Slice thickness
   d. kVp

24. Increasing mAs will decrease noise levels on the CT images. What will it do to patient dose?

   a. Decreases patient dose
   b. Does not affect patient dose
   c. Increases patient dose
   d. None of the above

25. What technical factor adapts the mA to the beam attenuation as a function of the projection angle allowing the current to be more efficient, thus reducing patient dose?

   a. MA modulation
   b. kVp
   c. Filtration
   d. Collimation

26. What is considered the most effective way to reduce the population dose from CT radiation exposure?

   a. Newer CT scanners
   b. Decrease the number of CT studies ordered
   c. Eliminate pediatric CT scans
   d. Iodine supplements

27. What are the two Scanner-Based radiation patient dose estimates displayed on the operator's console after the completion of a CT exam?

   a. MAs and kVp
   b. MSAD and DLP
   c. CTDI and DLP
   d. MAs and DLP

28. CTDIvol (CT Dose Index Volume) is a modified patient dose accounting for which technical parameter?

   a. Pitch
   b. Slice thickness
   c. Slice increment
   d. Filtration

29. Efforts and measures to reduce patient dose should be initiated by and are the responsibility of whom?

   a. Ordering physicians
   b. Clinical radiology staff
   c. CT manufacturers
   d. All of the above

30. Color coded weight based CT protocols have been developed for what population to help reduce patient dose?

    a. Geriatric
    b. Adult
    c. Pediatric
    d. All of the above

31. What process reduces the longest wave length photons creating a more monochromatic beam and reducing patient radiation dose?

    a. Filtration
    b. Detector collimation
    c. Slip rings
    d. None of the above

32. What component located within the CT Gantry measures transmitted photons that pass completely through the patient?

    a. Filters
    b. Detectors
    c. Collimators
    d. Slip rings

33. What is the most efficient and most common type of detector utilized today?

    a. Xenon gas detectors
    b. Stationary detectors
    c. Solid state crystalline detectors
    d. Single detectors

34. During Image Reconstruction in the Data Acquisition System, what system reconstructs the amplified digitized raw data into the CT images?

    a. Amplifier
    b. Analogue-to-digital converter (ADC)
    c. Array processor
    d. Operator's console

35. The development of what electromechanical device consisting of circular electrical conductive rings and brushes allowed for helical scanning capabilities?

    a. Amplifier
    b. Array processor
    c. Electron gun
    d. Slip rings

36. What CT development allows for more than one slice to be acquired during each tube rotation?

    a. Host computers
    b. Data acquisition system
    c. Multi-row detector arrays
    d. Single-row detector arrays

37. What is the component that takes a low voltage and passes it through a series of wire coils to produce a very large voltage?

   a. X-ray tube
   b. High voltage generator
   c. Low voltage generator
   d. Amplifier

38. What parameter determines the number of x-ray photons produced by the CT x-ray tube?

   a. MA
   b. KVp
   c. Slice thickness
   d. Table increment

39. What type of collimation restricts the x-ray beam immediately after it exits the CT tube and before any photons interact with a patient's body?

   a. Post-patient collimation
   b. Pre-detector collimation
   c. Pre-patient collimation
   d. All of the above

40. What system during Image Reconstruction in the Data Acquisition System makes the small energy or light emitted from the detectors larger?

   a. Amplifier
   b. Analogue-to-Digital Converter (ADC)
   c. Array processor
   d. Operator's console

41. CT generators produce high kV to increase the intensity and penetration of the beam. What is the general kV range?

   a. 140-170kV
   b. 60-120kV
   c. 40-150kV
   d. 120-140kV

42. What is the atomic number of Tungsten?

   a. 74
   b. 128
   c. 62
   d. 80

43. What are the most common size focal spots found in CT tubes?

   a. 1.0mm and 2.0mm
   b. 0.25mm and 1.0mm
   c. 0.5mm and 1.0mm
   d. 3.0mm and 4.25mm

44. What daily maintenance procedure is done to a group of low exposures to bring the tube temperature safely up to a proper operating temperature?

   a. Air calibrations
   b. Tube warm-up
   c. Gantry rotations
   d. Water phantom

45. During the Data Acquisition System process, where is the amplified signal converted to a digital form?

   a. Analogue-to-digital converter
   b. Amplified-to-digital converter
   c. Array processor
   d. Amplifier

46. What generation of CT scanners has a fixed anode, fan beam geometry, and linear detector array?

   a. 1st generation
   b. 2nd generation
   c. 3rd generation
   d. 4th generation

47. What generation of CT scanners has a rotating anode, fan beam geometry, multiple detector array along a curve, and the ability to provide helical scans?

   a. 1st generation
   b. 2nd generation
   c. 3rd generation
   d. 4th generation

48. What type of CT scanner has no x-ray tube and was the fastest cardiac CT scanner until MDCT?

   a. Cone beam CT
   b. Fluoroscopy CT
   c. Electron beam CT
   d. PET/CT scanners

49. The raw data from the array processor must be further processed to become the final CT image during what process?

   a. Filtered back projection
   b. Convolution
   c. Interpolation
   d. Modulation

50. What process occurs during image reconstruction that improves the image by applying a reconstruction filter or kernel to the data?

   a. Convolution
   b. Interpolation
   c. Cone beam reconstruction
   d. None of the above

51. What type of reconstruction filter minimizes the grainy appearance of the image?
   a. Sharp
   b. Smooth
   c. Both a and b
   d. None of the above

52. What type of data is obtained from the detector array and contains all the thousands of bits of data acquired with each scan?
   a. Image data
   b. Reconstructed data
   c. Helical data
   d. Raw data

53. What type of data is required for retrospective reconstruction?
   a. Reconstructed data
   b. Raw data
   c. Image data
   d. Retrospective data

54. The thickness of the slice that is actually represented on the CT image as opposed to the size selected by the collimator opening is called what?
   a. Volumetric slice thickness
   b. Serial slice thickness
   c. Effective slice thickness
   d. Selected slice thickness

55. What commonly adjusted imaging parameter determines where the helical slices will be reconstructed and if they will overlap or not?
   a. Reconstruction interval
   b. Scan FOV
   c. Reconstruction FOV
   d. Reconstruction filter

56. What post-processing technique reformats image data images acquired in one orientation or plane to images in other orientations or planes?
   a. Maximum Intensity Projection (MIP)
   b. Multi-planar reconstruction
   c. Retrospective reconstruction
   d. Volume rendering

57. What post-processing technique utilizes thin slices and overlapping helically acquired image data to reformat cross sectional anatomy to anatomical surface renderings?
   a. Retrospective surface rendering
   b. Slice misregistration
   c. Temporal resolution
   d. 3D surface rendering

58. What 3D technique selects voxels with the highest value to display as an image?
   a. Minimum-Intensity Projection (MinIP)
   b. Multi-planar Reformation (MPR)
   c. Modulation Transfer Function (MTF)
   d. Maximum-Intensity Projection (MIP)

59. The term defined as a two-dimensional square of data that when arranged in rows and columns makes up the image matrix is called what?
   a. Voxel
   b. Pixel
   c. CT number
   d. Hounsfield scale

60. What term defines a three dimensional cube of data acquired in CT or a volume element?
   a. Voxel
   b. Pixel
   c. CT number
   d. Image matrix

61. What plane axis determines the thickness of the slices?
   a. X-axis
   b. Y-axis
   c. Z-axis
   d. Q-axis

62. What is the field of view that covers the area within the gantry from which the raw data is acquired?
   a. Scan field of view (SFOV)
   b. Reconstruction field of view (RFOV)
   c. Display field of view (DFOV)
   d. None of the above

63. Increasing the reconstruction FOV will have what effect on patient dose?
   a. Increases
   b. No effect
   c. Decreases
   d. Depends on the image matrix size

64. The size of the pixels equals the reconstruction FOV divided by what?
   a. Matrix
   b. Voxels
   c. SFOV
   d. Y-coordinates

65. What term describes adjusting the brightness and contrast of the gray shades assigned to represent the tissues in the pixels of a CT image?

   a. Magnification
   b. ROI
   c. Linearity
   d. Windowing

66. What post-processed image adjustment to the final displayed image determines the range of CT numbers that occupy the full gray scale?

   a. Window level
   b. Window width
   c. Image magnification
   d. Image resolution

67. Who is generally recognized as the inventor of computerized tomography?

   a. A.M. Cormack
   b. W.C. Roentgen
   c. G.N. Hounsfield
   d. W.A. Kalender

68. What two systems exhibit negative CT values due to their lower density and therefore lower attenuation coefficient?

   a. Lung tissue and fat
   b. Muscle and bone
   c. Contrast media and bone
   d. Fat and calcium

69. What archiving and communication system provides rapid retrieval of images, cost-effective storage, multiple modality image access, and a secure network for patient data transmission?

   a. PACS
   b. DICOM
   c. PDF
   d. RIS

70. What is considered the universally accepted standard for the transferal of radiologic images and other medical information between computers and across geographical locations?

   a. NEMA
   b. DICOM
   c. PACS
   d. Host computer

71. Are PACS systems required to comply with HIPAA regulations?

   a. No
   b. Yes
   c. Varies by state
   d. Varies by facility

72. What are the acceptable methods of medical image archival and back-up storage required in the United States by the Security Rules Administrative Safeguards section of HIPAA?

   a. Hard drive copy
   b. Optical media
   c. Magnetic tape
   d. All of the above

73. What type of archiving utilized storage devices, such as hard drives, are instantly accessible to the user?

   a. Online archiving
   b. Off-line archiving
   c. Optical disc libraries
   d. None of the above

74. Electronic interference that causes the image to appear grainy due to insufficient photon numbers is called what?

   a. Resolution
   b. Beam hardening
   c. Noise
   d. Tube arcing

75. What term is used to describe the ability to differentiate small differences in density where the photon energy level plays a key role in the image outcome?

   a. Resolution
   b. Contrast
   c. Noise
   d. Pitch

76. Often expressed in terms of line pairs in CT, what is a measurement of the smallest visualized structure in the image?

   a. Resolution
   b. Contrast
   c. Noise
   d. Pitch

77. What term describes the ability of the scanner to produce the same CT number regardless of the ROI location within a homogeneous object?

   a. Noise
   b. Spatial resolution
   c. Temporal resolution
   d. Uniformity

78. The speed that the CT image data can be acquired is important to reduce or eliminate artifacts that occur from object motion. What is this acquired speed called?

   a. Spatial resolution
   b. Temporal resolution
   c. Uniformity
   d. Table speed

79. Temporal Resolution is determined by three things: the gantry rotation, the speed with which the system can record changing signals, and
   a. Patient habitus
   b. Reconstruction algorithms
   c. Number of detector channels
   d. Slice thickness accuracy

80. What is assigned to represent the attenuation properties of the tissues in each pixel?
   a. Voxels
   b. Gray scale
   c. Matrix
   d. CT number

81. Which window center and window width would best display a lung window at the viewing console?
   a. C/W -50, 400
   b. C/W -600, 1700
   c. C/W 1000, 2500
   d. C/W 700, -2000

82. What is a property of the CT system characterized by output that is directly proportional to input, and describes the amount to which the CT number of an object is proportional to the actual object density in HU?
   a. Linearity
   b. Convolution
   c. Interpolation
   d. Line pairs

83. What device is used for quality assurance to evaluate a broad range of scanning parameters including both spatial and contrast resolution?
   a. Laser lights
   b. Phantoms
   c. Ionization chamber
   d. Windmill

84. Which common artifact occurs when there's an increase in the average energy of the x-ray beam as it penetrates tissue causing dark bands or streaks through the CT image?
   a. Beam hardening
   b. Partial volume
   c. Ring
   d. Motion

85. Which of the following will help minimize beam hardening artifacts?
   a. Correction algorithms
   b. Thinner slices
   c. Avoid scanning through very dense contrast
   d. All of the above

86. What is the common artifact that appears as blurriness or incorrect CT numbers causing pathology to be missed or misdiagnosed, and which fails to appear on all views?

   a. Beam hardening
   b. Partial volume averaging
   c. Metal
   d. Motion

87. What hardware related artifact is caused by a faulty or miscalibrated detector element?

   a. Metal artifact
   b. Streak artifact
   c. Ring artifact
   d. Cone beam artifact

88. Tube arching is a common equipment induced artifact caused by a surge of what?

   a. Electrical current
   b. Photons
   c. Gantry rotation
   d. Detector energy

89. Which artifact produces streaking or light and dark shading due to scanning irregular shaped objects that contain a pronounced difference in density from the surrounding tissues?

   a. Beam hardening
   b. Edge gradient effect
   c. Patient positioning
   d. Cone beam

90. Routine brain CT scans should end at the vertex and begin where?

   a. Skull base
   b. Orbits
   c. Vomer
   d. Zygoma

91. What is the preferred modality used to image the posterior fossa?

   a. CT
   b. MRI
   c. PET scan
   d. X-ray

92. When scanning Internal Auditory Canals (Temporal Bones) what indication requires IV contrast?

   a. Cholesteatoma
   b. Mastoiditis
   c. Acoustic neuroma
   d. Ear infections

93. What gland lies within the sella of the sphenoid bone and is usually imaged with IV contrast?
   a. Clinoid
   b. Pituitary
   c. Thymus
   d. Medulla

94. The axial images on an orbit CT scan best visualize the Lateral Rectus Muscles and what?
   a. Optic nerve
   b. Mastoid air cells
   c. Auricle
   d. Orbital roof

95. In order to better visualize air fluid levels within the sinuses, the patient should be scanned in what position?
   a. Supine
   b. Feet first
   c. Prone
   d. Head first

96. A patient presents to the Emergency Room with severe facial trauma. Which criteria below is the best possible Maxillofacial CT protocol?
   a. Helical/1.25mm slices/coronals/axials
   b. Prone/5mm slices/coronals
   c. Supine/1.25mm slices/axials
   d. Prone/2mm slices/standard algorithm

97. What indication recommends that IV contrast be administered during an Orbital CT scan?
   a. Trauma
   b. Grave's disease
   c. Foreign body
   d. Cellulitis

98. What head CT protocol is usually always scanned serial/conventional rather than helical for fine detail and the best image quality possible?
   a. Routine brain
   b. CTA brain
   c. Orbits
   d. Maxillofacial

99. What CT Head exam's quality is strictly dependent on matching the time windows for contrast enhancement and starting the scan?
   a. Pituitary
   b. CTA COW
   c. IAC's
   d. TMJ's

100. To help reduce radiation exposure to the lens of the eyes it is recommended to program the CT slices of a routine brain CT parallel to what?

   a. Orbital meatal line
   b. Zygomatic arch
   c. Frontal sinuses
   d. Supraorbital meatal line

101. The dense bones of the skull produce what common artifact while imaging the posterior fossa?

   a. Beam hardening
   b. Partial volume averaging
   c. Metal
   d. Motion

102. What medication must be administered within 3 hours of the first signs of a stroke to reverse disability?

   a. Aspirin
   b. Coumadin
   c. t-PA
   d. None of the above

103. What standard window settings are used for a trauma brain for bone windows?

   a. 160/40
   b. 2500/400
   c. -2000/500
   d. 200/60

104. IV contrast is usually indicated when scanning the neck except for which indications?

   a. Foreign body
   b. Salivary duct stone
   c. Scheduled iodine therapy for thyroid
   d. All of the above

105. During a CT scan of the neck, having the patient not swallow during image acquisition will help to do what?

   a. Stop patient from choking
   b. Minimize PVA
   c. Relax neck vasculature
   d. Minimize motion

106. Bolus timing for Soft Tissue Neck CT's can be difficult due to many different structures enhancing at varied times. What contrast injection technique helps address the contradictory timing goals for imaging the neck?

   a. Split bolus
   b. Venous and arterial scans
   c. Decrease injection rate
   d. Increase delay times

107. What imaging modality is considered the "gold standard" for the imaging of cerebrovascular disorders?

   a. MR angiography
   b. CT angiography
   c. Interventional angiography
   d. None of the above

108. What is the most common neck site where TIA's originate?

   a. Jugular
   b. Carotid
   c. Basilar
   d. Vertebral

109. What imaging modality provides fast and accurate diagnosis (and therefore treatment) of post-laryngeal trauma?

   a. Endoscopy
   b. Ultrasound
   c. MRI
   d. CT

110. A routine Chest CT to stage or question lung cancer begins at the sternal notch and ends with what anatomy?

   a. Liver
   b. Lungs
   c. Adrenal glands
   d. T-12

111. When imaging the chest for CT of the airways, what breathing technique should be utilized?

   a. Inspiration
   b. Expiration
   c. Both A and B
   d. None of the above

112. What chest CT protocol should be done to evaluate the lung parenchyma in patients with known or suspected lung diseases like emphysema and fibrosis?

   a. High-resolution CT (HRCT)
   b. CTA chest
   c. Routine chest CT with lung windows
   d. Soft tissue neck with routine chest CT

113. The contrast media follows the systemic circulation of the body. Where does the contrast flow to after it leaves the Superior Vena Cava (SVC)?

   a. Subclavian artery
   b. Right heart atrium
   c. Left heart ventricle
   d. Aorta

114. After imaging the arterial system for thrombosis, what may be performed to assess venous thrombosis in the pelvis and/or lower extremities?

   a. CTA run-off
   b. CT venography
   c. CT lower extremities
   d. Routine pelvic CT

115. What two techniques are utilized during Cardiac CTA to improve motion artifact from the beating heart muscle?

   a. Patient immobilization and beta blockers
   b. Beta blockers and cardiac gating
   c. Cardiac gating and nitroglycerin
   d. Hydration and rest

116. CTA Chest protocols for the evaluation of Pulmonary Emboli scanned in which manner will help to minimize respiratory motion artifacts?

   a. Caudal-cranial
   b. Cranial-caudal
   c. Direction of scan will not impact respiration motion
   d. Thicker slices to reduce length of scan

117. What is considered crucial to creating a diagnostic CTA examination of the Chest when it comes to contrast media?

   a. Contrast dose
   b. Contrast timing
   c. Contrast rate
   d. All of the above

118. Why is a power injected saline flush recommended after the injection of contrast media for CTA pulmonary studies?

   a. Reduces beam-hardening artifacts
   b. Reduces patient radiation attenuation
   c. Increases partial volume averaging
   d. Increases image acquisition speed

119. How has the development of multi-detector CT improved thoracic imaging?

   a. Improved spatial and temporal resolution
   b. Higher mA and kVp limits
   c. Decreased tube cooling times
   d. MDCT advances did not improve thoracic imaging

120. What laboratory test plays a valuable role in the workup for possible Pulmonary Embolism?

   a. PTT
   b. Creatinine
   c. D-Dimer
   d. BUN

121. The pulmonary artery closely follows what anatomical structure thus making it easy to identify on cross-sectional imaging?

    a. Ascending aorta
    b. Sternum
    c. Trachea
    d. Bronchial tree

122. What is one good reason for scanning a HR Chest CT in the prone position?

    a. Better spatial resolution
    b. Demonstrate densities affected by gravity
    c. More comfortable for the patient
    d. Never scan a HR chest CT prone

123. What imaging plane is displayed in the below Brain CT?

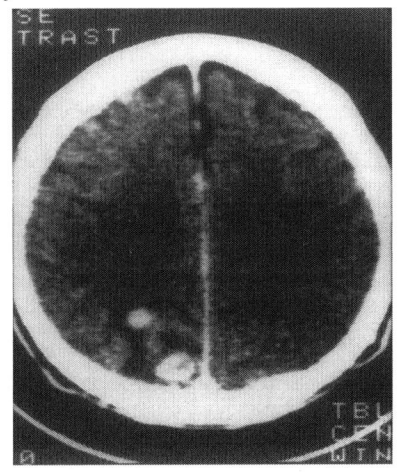

    a. Sagittal
    b. Axial
    c. Coronal
    d. Oblique

124. What imaging plane is displayed on the below Sinus CT image?

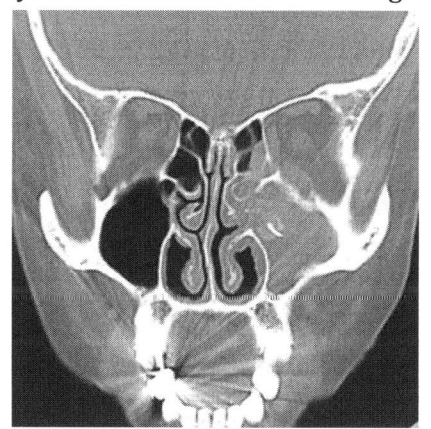

   a. Sagittal
   b. Axial
   c. Coronal
   d. Oblique

125. What anatomy is represented on letter B?

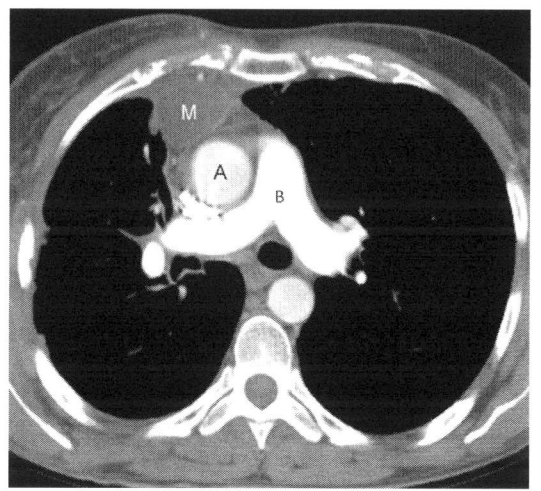

   a. Aorta
   b. Main pulmonary artery
   c. IVC
   d. Pulmonary vein

126. What imaging plane is displayed on the below Cervical Spine CT image?

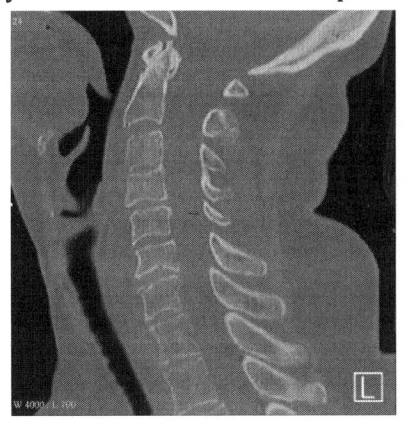

a. Sagittal
b. Axial
c. Coronal
d. Oblique

127. What are the two phases of the Non-Equilibrium Phase utilized for Bi-Phasic studies of the pancreas and liver?

a. Hepatic arterial and portal venous
b. Bolus and equilibrium
c. Hepatic arterial and bolus
d. Portal venous and equilibrium

128. What is the least optimal volume of the oral contrast agent for the best possible bowel opacification?

a. 200 mL
b. 300 mL
c. 600 mL
d. 100 mL

129. What is the best reason for utilizing oral contrast to opacify the GI tract?

a. Distention of the GI tract
b. Differentiates fluid filled bowel from a mass or abscess
c. Evacuates feces for a clean GI tract
d. Evaluates the lymph system

130. What window width and level setting adequately displays most soft tissue abdominal anatomy?

a. 2000/600
b. 1500/-600
c. 450/50
d. 150/70

131. What liver pathology is displayed as a well-defined, hypo-dense mass on an unenhanced image, and after contrast enhancement progressively enhances along the periphery and eventually is uniformly enhanced?
    a. Fatty infiltration
    b. Hemangioma
    c. Tumorous mass
    d. Liver cyst

132. CT is the imaging modality of choice for what abdominal organ?
    a. Pancreas
    b. Gallbladder
    c. Large intestines
    d. Stomach

133. What protocol would be utilized to get the most information about the kidneys, ureters, and bladders?
    a. CT pelvis
    b. CT abdomen
    c. CT urography
    d. Ultrasound

134. Typically, scan delay time for a portal venous phase of the liver is between
    a. 75-85 seconds.
    b. 10-20 seconds.
    c. 25-30 seconds.
    d. 65-75 seconds.

135. What is the appropriate contrast protocol to diagnose urinary tract calculi?
    a. Barium sulfate only
    b. No oral and no IV contrast
    c. IV contrast only
    d. Oral and IV contrast

136. A routine liver abdomen CT is often scanned is one portal venous phase. What is an indication to scan the liver bi-phasic?
    a. Hyper-vascular lesions
    b. Hepatic vascular anatomy
    c. Hemangiomas
    d. All of the above

137. What abdominal organ's masses are diagnosed benign or malignant based on their attenuation values and the degree of contrast wash out on delayed imaging?
    a. Pancreas
    b. Adrenals
    c. Spleen
    d. Gallbladder

138. The average scan delay time for IV contrast helical CT imaging of the spleen is
    a. 75-85 seconds.
    b. 10-20 seconds.
    c. 25-30 seconds.
    d. 65-75 seconds.

139. Peak intravascular enhancement is necessary for all CTA exams. What criteria below will ensure a CTA of the Aorta will produce great images?
    a. 18G IV access
    b. Dense contrast material over 300
    c. Injection rate of 5cc/sec.
    d. All of the above

140. What is a typical mAs used in routine abdomen CT studies on an average sized patient?
    a. 400-500 mAs
    b. 25-100 mAs
    c. 200-300 mAs
    d. 100-150 mAs

141. What method or type of contrast administration may occur if the distal colon is not properly opacified with timed oral contrast agents for a Pelvic CT exam?
    a. IV contrast
    b. Cystografin
    c. Rectal contrast
    d. Intrathecal contrast

142. What is the typical gantry tilt for a routine Pelvic CT?
    a. 30 degrees
    b. -30 degrees
    c. 15 degrees
    d. No tilt

143. What are the proper anatomical imaging parameters utilized during a routine Pelvic CT exam?
    a. Iliac crests through symphysis pubis
    b. Above the diaphragm through the symphysis pubis
    c. Above the diaphragm through the iliac crests
    d. Iliac crests through knees

144. What vessels begin after the abdominal aorta bifurcates at around the level of L-4?
    a. Common iliac arteries
    b. Femoral arteries
    c. Carotid arteries
    d. Celiac arteries

145. What anatomy is displayed below on letter A?

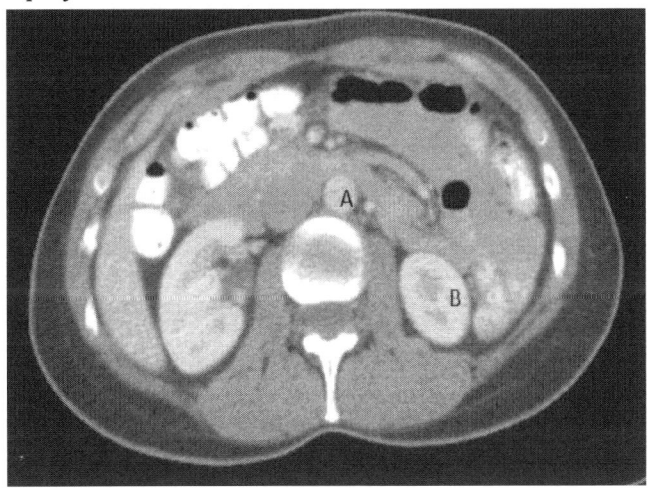

a. Kidney
b. Adrenal gland
c. Pancreas
d. Aorta

146. What anatomy is displayed below on letter B?

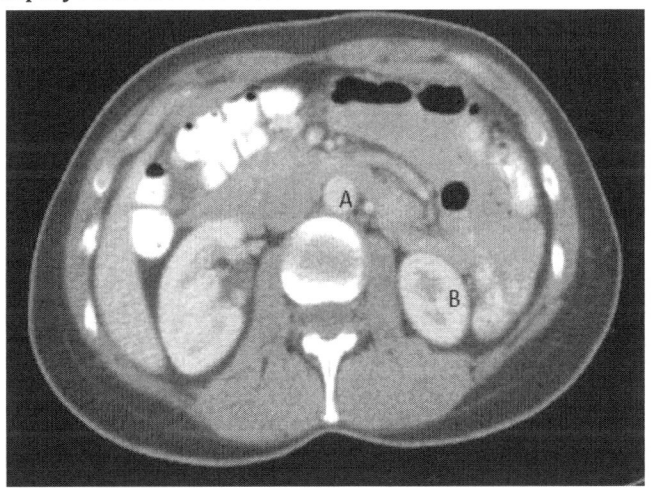

a. Kidney
b. Adrenal gland
c. Pancreas
d. Aorta

147. What anatomy is displayed below on letter A?

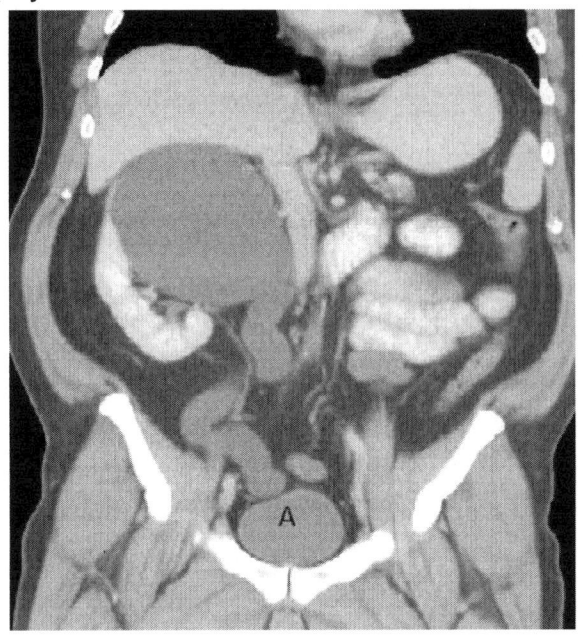

a. Uterus
b. Bladder
c. Prostate
d. Appendix

148. McBurney's sign is a common exam that is used to help diagnose what classic disease process?

a. Pancreatitis
b. Abdominal aneurysm
c. Appendicitis
d. Leukocytosis

149. A dilated non-opacified appendix with soft tissue stranding commonly represents what diagnosis?

a. Acute appendicitis
b. Ruptured appendix
c. Normal appendix
d. Appendicolith

150. What is the average volume of IV contrast utilized for a routine Abdomen and Pelvic CT exam?

a. 25-50 cc
b. 65-100 cc
c. 150-200 cc
d. 200-250cc

151. What are the best patient positioning factors when scanning a routine Abdomen and Pelvic CT?

a. Head first, prone, arms down
b. Feet first, supine, arms down
c. Head first, supine, arms over head
d. Feet first, supine, arms over head

152. What would the likely diagnosis be on a homogenous adrenal mass with an attenuation number on an unenhanced CT of less than 10 HU?
   a. Adenoma
   b. Primary adrenal carcinoma
   c. Adrenal metastasis
   d. Normal adrenal gland tissue

153. What vessel is represented by letter A on the image below?

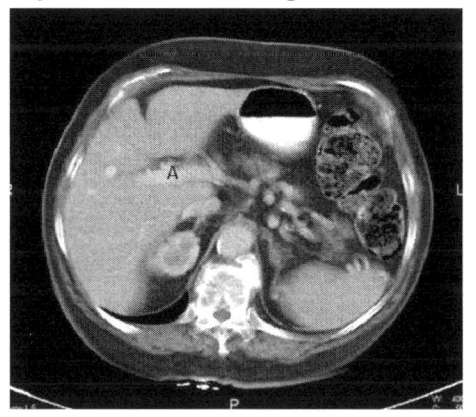

   a. Celiac vein
   b. Portal vein
   c. Renal artery
   d. Splenic vein

154. It is ideal when scanning long bones of the musculoskeletal system that the plane of the CT section is _____ to the long axis of the bone.
   a. Parallel
   b. Oblique
   c. Perpendicular
   d. At 30 degree angle

155. When a patient is positioned for a foot/ankle CT in the gantry with their toes pointing straight up with no gantry angle, on what plane is data acquired?
   a. Oblique coronal plane
   b. Direct axial plane
   c. Coronal plane
   d. Direct sagittal plane

156. When the scan plane is perpendicular to the subtalar joint and the gantry is tilted towards the patient at around 25 degrees, what is the directly acquired imaging plane?
   a. Oblique coronal plane
   b. Direct axial plane
   c. Coronal plane
   d. Direct sagittal plane

157. CT arthrography of the shoulder is useful for evaluating loose bodies within the joint and what structure(s)?

a. Scapula
b. Sternoclavicular joint
c. Joint capsule and intracapsular structures
d. Humerus and glenoid bones

158. What is the proper delay time to scan a post myelogram patient after the injection of intrathecal contrast has been administered?

a. Less than 30 minutes
b. 1-3 hours
c. 4-5 hours
d. Immediately

159. When the soft tissues (cartilage, ligaments, and muscles) of any extremity need to be evaluated, what is the imaging modality of choice?

a. CT
b. PET
c. X-Ray
d. MRI

160. What is the optimal scan slice thickness when imaging all musculoskeletal anatomy?

a. 5mm-7.5mm
b. 0.625mm-1.25mm
c. 2mm-3mm
d. 10mm

161. What anatomy is depicted below for letter A?

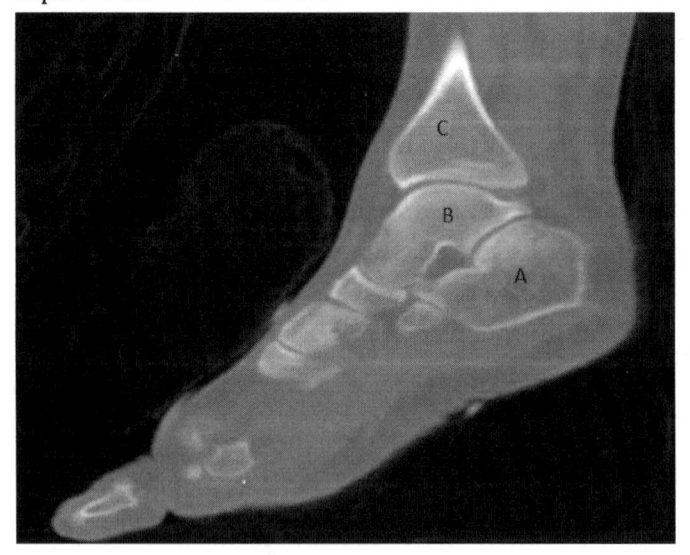

a. Calcaneus
b. Fibula
c. Talus
d. Tibia

162. What anatomy is depicted below for letter A?

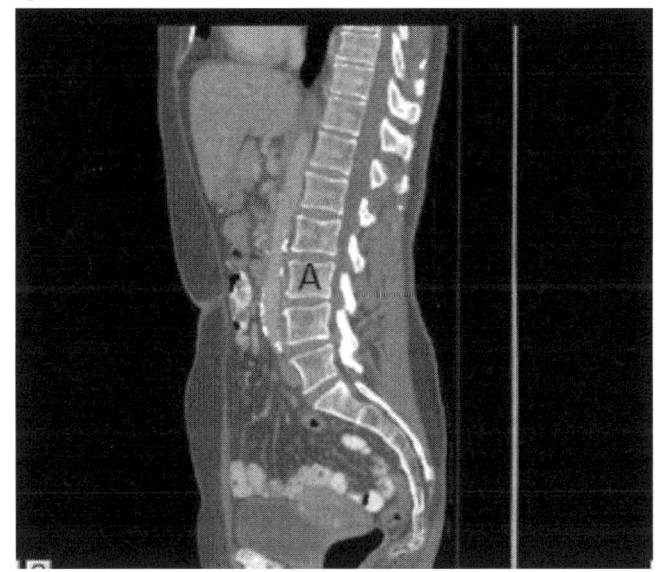

a. L-2
b. L-3
c. T-1
d. L-4

163. What anatomy is depicted below for letter A?

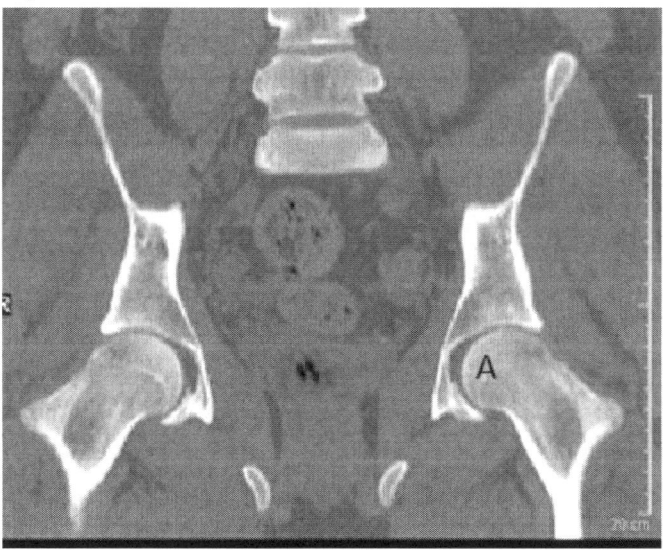

a. Femoral head
b. Iliac crest
c. Pubis
d. Ischium

164. What anatomy is depicted below for letter A?

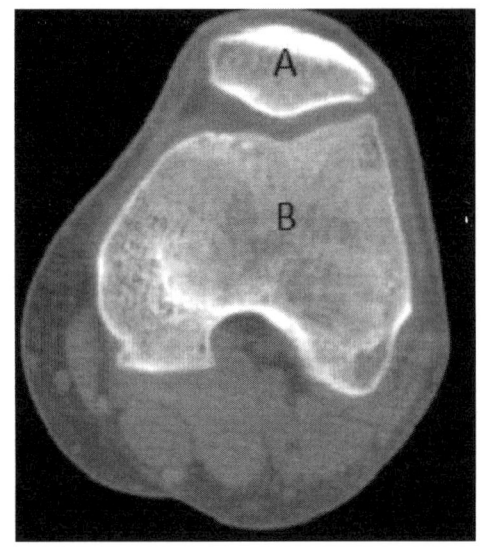

a. Medial femoral condyle
b. Popliteal
c. Patella
d. Tibial plateau

165. What anatomy is depicted below for letter A?

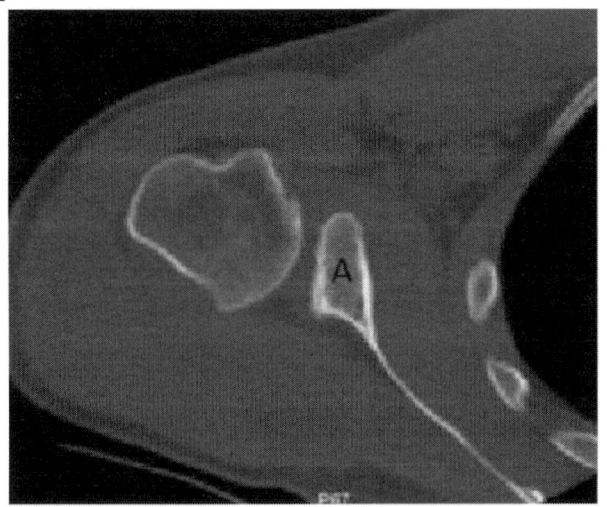

a. Scapula
b. Iliac crest
c. Humeral head
d. Sternum

Answer Key and Explanations

1. **D:** It is important to always ask women of child bearing age if there is any chance of pregnancy prior to any CT exam. If there is a chance, a pregnancy test needs to be negative prior to scanning the patient. All patients should be asked about allergies prior to a CT scan. The patient may have a latex allergy or a known IV contrast reaction history. Diabetes can affect a patient's renal function, so lab work may be required prior to an IV contrast injection to make sure the kidneys can excrete the contrast from the blood. Also, certain diabetic medications also affect renal function. These medications may need to be stopped before and/or after IV contrast injections until renal function tests are performed. All these pre-screening questions should be asked again by the CT technologist immediately prior to the scan.

2. **D:** There are many variations of consent forms available that vary by state and by facility. Signed consent forms are required at some facilities prior to administering IV contrast during a CT scan. This is done to prove that the patient was informed about the risks and side effects and still agrees to have the contrast injection. There are currently no universal laws that mandate a signed informed consent.

3. **D:** Many patients are apprehensive about getting a CT scan. When a patient knows exactly what to expect they usually feel less anxious and are able to follow the scan instructions. Proper pre-scan preparations with oral prep, NPO instructions, and dress attire will minimize the risk for needing portions of the exam or even the entire procedure to be repeated thus reducing radiation dose to the patient and attaining the best possible images for that patient.

4. **A:** BUN and Creatinine levels indicate the ability of the patient's renal systems to clear the contrast media from the blood. The BUN provides information about the ability of the kidneys to remove impurities from the blood. Elevated Creatinine levels indicate an impairment of the ability of the kidneys to excrete creatinine from the blood. Renal Disease impairs the ability of the kidneys to remove impurities from the blood. IV Contrast Media is considered an impurity and can cause a nephrotoxic effect in the patient. It is important to pre-screen most patients prior to administering IV contrast to ensure that they can clear the contrast from their blood.

5. **C:** Every facility interprets the normal range somewhat differently, but these are typical normal ranges. Urea is a waste product produced in the breakdown of protein in the liver, released in the bloodstream, filtered in the kidneys, and excreted in urine. When the kidneys are not properly working, there is a rise in blood urea nitrogen. Many other things can affect BUN levels such as certain medications, high protein foods, age, sex, dehydration, and pregnancy.

6. **C:** If the patient is having any kind of interventional procedure with CT Guidance, lab tests to determine the blood's ability to coagulate need to be done. The imaging staff need to be sure that the patient's blood has the correct clotting ability so the patient doesn't bleed internally. Such procedures may include all types of CT Guided Biopsies of any area, CT Guided drainages, and Ablations. If the PT or PTT are abnormal, the procedure may be cancelled.

7. **B:** Aseptic technique is a method that prevents the introduction of unwanted organisms into an environment that may cause an infection. Nosocomial infections are common in hospitals, and it is the medical staff that is responsible for lowering the incidence of hospital acquired infections. Anytime the skin is broken, a chance of infection is possible. Aseptic technique helps to prevent infection. Hand washing, gloves, sterile supplies, and proper skin preparation are all a part of utilizing an aseptic technique for peripheral IV access.

8. A: CT Angiograms are scanning the patient during the Bolus or Arterial phase of the IV contrast injection. Faster scanners also require faster injection times. Peripheral venous access with a smaller needle will not safely allow the technologist to inject the contrast at an optimal rate to catch the arterial phase. In addition to the size of the needle, the site should be anti-cubital and proximal. Certain mid-lines are rated for the contrast injection rate and PSI that are needed for a CTA injection. These specific catheters must be documented in the patient chart.

9. B: Enhancement times are directly related to injection rate, volume of contrast media, velocity of blood flow, and patient cardiac output. The first phase of enhancement is the Bolus phase. This is an optimal phase for CTAs. There is a significant density difference between the abdominal aorta and IVC. The second phase is the Non-Equilibrium phase. During this phase, the bolus disperses into the capillaries then into the veins. The two phases of enhancement within this phase are the Hepatic Arterial and Portal Venous. The Non-Equilibrium phase provides the best differentiation of structures in soft tissue like the liver and pancreas. The third phase is Equilibrium. During this phase, the concentration of contrast in the veins and arteries are similar and soft tissue differentiation becomes diminished.

10. D: If the IV manufacturer of a .22 gauge needle is only rated for a certain rate and PSI, the technologist must adhere to those limitations. Injecting too fast through a smaller needle catheter may cause an infiltration or cause the injector to stop the injection due to pressure limiting. The type of CT exam will also determine the flow rate. A CT Angiogram will require a faster rate and a soft tissue neck will require a slower rate. A 64 slice scanner will scan much faster than a 4 slice CT scanner. The technologist may miss a particular necessary diagnosing phase if these factors are not taken into consideration while selecting a proper flow rate.

11. C: Known or suspected GI perforation, colon obstruction, pyloric stenosis, and known barium allergy are also contraindications to administering Barium Sulfate. If Barium Sulfate is aspirated into the lungs it can cause aspiration pneumonitis. Barium Sulfate is also caustic to the retroperitoneal cavity if it was leaking out of the GI tract from a perforation. Barium Sulfate is used if a patient has an allergy to Iodine.

12. A: Osmolality refers to the number of particles in a solution. Ionic contrast agents break into the charges particles in the bloodstream, and Non-Ionic contrast agents remain intact. The osmolality of blood ranges from 280-303 mOmg/kg, whereas Ionic contrast rages from 1300-1600 mOmg/kg. This causes an obvious reaction within the body. Ionic contrasts have a higher reaction and death rate but are inexpensive.

13. C: Contrast Media is used in CT to improve the sensitivity and specificity of clinical diagnoses. Barium Sulfate, Gastrografin, and IV contrast agents are all positive contrast agents. They are attenuated by the x-ray beam, so they show as a density. A negative contrast agent is not attenuated by the x-ray beam. Air is used as a negative contrast agent during virtual CT colonoscopies. Water is also used to dilate the GI tract without presenting an attenuated density.

14. C: Osmolality refers to the number of particles in a solution. The osmolality of blood ranges from 280-303 mOmg/kg, and iso-osmolar contrast is the same or less than blood. It is more expensive, but it is much gentler on the kidneys. The patient also feels fewer side effects. Asthma, renal insufficiencies, and highly anxious patients benefit from iso-osmolar contrast agents.

15. B: Imaging locations vary by type and volume, but rectal contrast is often used to enhance the large intestines and pelvic organs. The rectal contrast helps to increase the sensitivity of the CT exam by outlining the large intestines, bladder, uterus, prostate and other organs. Rectal contrast is

utilized for rectal pathology, or when a patient has lower GI symptoms but cannot tolerate oral prep. The contrast may be given using an enema tip attached to a bag or inserted manually using a tip and syringes.

16. C: Pheochromocytoma is a rare (usually benign) tumor of adrenal gland tissue. It results in the release of too much epinephrine and norepinephrine, hormones that control heart rate, metabolism, and blood pressure. An injection of IV Contrast material in patients with this condition can invoke a hypertensive crisis, so in most cases it is a contraindication to IV contrast injections. If it is approved by the Radiologist and imperative to the CT exam, careful blood pressure monitoring before during and after the CT contrast injection will be crucial.

17. A: Multiple Myeloma is a malignant bone condition that can cause kidney failure, abnormal proteins in the plasma, and abnormal urine proteins. IV contrast may cause the proteins to precipitate, resulting in renal obstruction and possibly renal failure. Multiple Myeloma becomes a true risk for nephrotoxicity when there is pre-existing renal insufficiency present. Each imaging facility maintains protocols on this condition as it relates to IV contrast injections.

18. D: Minor Reactions to contrast would include minor hives, headache, itching, shaking, sweating, nausea/vomiting, and dizziness. Moderate Reactions include hypertension, hypotension, bronchospasm, facial edema, moderate hives, and wheezing. A Delayed Reaction occurs 30 plus minutes after the injection of IV contrast and usually before 7 days post injection. The Delayed Reaction can include fatigue, rash, headache, and flu-like symptoms. A Severe Reaction to the injection of IV contrast is rare, but it will include myocardial infarction, seizures, and respiratory arrest.

19. D: The increased speed capabilities of newer helical CT scanners require the IV contrast to be injected at a faster rate. The injection rate affects patient tolerance. Studies show that a faster injection increases adverse reactions in the patient. The total volume injected will also increase the risk of adverse reactions. A higher iodine concentration creates better enhancement on the CT images due to more attenuation. It also leads to a higher dose of contrast. A higher concentration of iodine has a higher osmolality therefore leading to increased incidence of adverse reactions.

20. A: Viscosity determines a fluids resistance to flow. More force is required to inject a more viscous contrast agent. Reduced viscosity will increase patient comfort at the injection site, decrease the risk of extravasations, and allow for a faster injection rate. Faster injection rates are required for newer helical CT scanners and all angiogram studies. Contrast viscosity is reduced by warming the agent to body temperature. Most CT suites have a warming box, and the power injector units have a warming sleeve to keep the contrast warm.

21. C: Intrathecal contrast agents are injected through the theca of the spinal cord into the subarachnoid space during a spine myelogram by a Radiologist or other Physician. The contrast agent must be a non-ionic, water-soluble, radiographic agent indicated for intrathecal administration. Misadministration of ionic contrast media can result in spasms and convulsions that will often lead to death. CT is often utilized post myelogram to further diagnostic findings. The CT scan should be done before 4 hours post injection or the contrast density will be too reduced. Some facilities have the patient roll to mix the contrast media and CSF or scan the patient prone.

22. D: Metformin (Glucophage) is a diabetic medication used to treat Type 2 Diabetes. It helps control the amount of sugar present in the blood. Iodinated contrast agents can cause an acute decline in renal function when injected intravenously. This may place a patient taking Metformin at a higher than normal risk for lactic acidosis. Lactic acidosis is a serious metabolic complication that

can occur due to Metformin accumulation. It can be fatal. Every facility maintains a Metformin protocol/policy to follow that usually instructs patients to stop taking their Metformin 24 hours prior to CT scan and 48 hours after CT scan. Renal function lab tests are done to make sure the kidneys are excreting properly before the patient can resume taking Metformin. A low osmolar, non-ionic contrast is safer for all diabetic patients.

23. A: Pitch is the distance in millimeters the table moves during one rotation of the x-ray tube divided by the slice thickness for single-row detectors. For MDCT, pitch equals the distance in millimeters the table moves during one rotation of the x-ray tube divided by the total slice volume or the thickness of a single slice. Pitch affects how quickly we can scan a large distance of anatomy. Increasing Pitch provides more anatomical coverage in less time, rapid coverage for CTAs, faster scanning times for trauma patients, and decreases the radiation dose. Decreasing Pitch will minimize noise, improve resolution, and increase patient radiation dose. It is considered one of the most important parameters in helical scanning.

24. C: The mathematical product of mA (tube current) and the 360 degree tube rotation time is mAs. Patient dose is directly related to mAs. Increasing mAs will decrease noise and increase patient dose. Fine anatomical detail is visualized when the noise level is less. Changing the mAs will have no direct effect on the CT image contrast or resolution.

25. A: Traditionally, the mA in CT is kept constant throughout the exam. This is technically simple, but it is an inefficient method of utilizing mA. Tube current modulation adapts the tube current to the beam attenuation from the localizers or real time scans. It allows the available x-ray power to be utilized more efficiently. Patient dose can be greatly reduced using mA modulation without affecting image quality.

26. B: When a CT scan is justified my medical necessity, the radiation risk is small relative to the diagnostic results obtained. However, there are a significant number of CT exams that are not justified by medical need. Children are often irradiated without convincing medical need. Patients and Physicians need to be educated on the radiation risks versus the benefits. This will help control the overall population radiation dose from medical ionizing radiation.

27. C: CT Dose Index (CTDI) and Dose Length Product (DLP) are two related measures of CT radiation dose available on CT consoles. CTDI is the primary dose measurement in CT. It denotes the average absorbed dose, along the z axis, from a series of contiguous exposures. It is measured from one axial CT scan (one rotation of the x-ray tube), and is calculated by dividing the absorbed dose by the total beam width. Several variations of the CTDI have been defined over the years. DLP is the CTDI multiplied by the scan length (slice thickness × number of slices) in centimeters. DLP is independent of what is actually scanned. The reported DLP is the same whether a small infant or a large child is scanned if the scan length and other scan parameters are the same. DLP is only an approximation of dose.

28. A: CTDI is a measurement interpreted as dose from the one scanned slice that would result from an entire procedure with continuous slices. CTDI is used by the FDA and CT manufacturers. CTDIw is a weighted average of CTDI as a standard single number descriptor of patient radiation dose from a CT scan. Helical scan capabilities required another method of calculation and technical factors to consider (such as the z axis). CTDIvol accounts for the pitch. CTDIw represents the average absorbed radiation dose over the x and y directions, and CTDIvol represents the average absorbed radiation dose over the x, y and z directions. Pitch is the most important parameter in helical scanning, and it determines the volume covered, image quality, and radiation exposure to the patient. CTDIvol= CTDIw/Pitch

29. D: It is the ordering physician's responsibility to make sure their patients' symptoms necessitate a CT exam. The clinical radiology staff is responsible for selecting the proper protocol based on the patient's individual history and the appropriate technical factors to get the best possible images and the least possible dose (ALARA principle). The manufacturers of CT equipment are responsible for developing dose-efficient systems together with special technical measures.

30. C: The pediatric population is the most sensitive to the effects of ionizing radiation. CT manufacturers and Radiology professionals developed color coded weight based protocol selections to help reduce the pediatric population radiation dose per CT exam. These color coded protocols will help the technologist select a protocol with tailored technical parameters for a patient's size/weight.

31. A: Filtration helps a polychromatic beam become monochromatic. It reduces the longest wave lengths or lower energy wave lengths. Thus the radiation dose to the patient is reduced without a significant decrease in the measured signal. The remaining x-rays are less prone to beam hardening and artifacts caused by beam hardening.

32. B: Detectors are located within the Gantry of the CT unit. They measure the transmitted photons that pass completely through the patient from the x-ray tube. They convert the photons to electrical signals by measuring attenuation. For an x-ray photon to generate a signal, it must enter the detector, collide with the detector atom, and produce a measurable event of electricity or light. The measureable light or energy from the detectors is a very small electrical signal that must be processed through the Data Acquisition System (DAS) to be amplified and made into an actual CT image. First Generation CT Scanners contain a single detector. Second Generation Scanners contain a linear detector array or a group of detectors in a straight line. The Third Generation Scanners contain a multiple detector array along a curve with complete circular rotation of detectors. Fourth Generation Scanners contain a rotating fan beam within a stationary ring of detectors. The development of Multi-Row Detector Scanners or MDCT provided the ability to collect information from multiple anatomical slices for each tube rotation. This allowed for faster scans, increased anatomical coverage, and thinner slices. MDCT utilizes Third Generation technology with multiple parallel detector arrays.

33. C: The most common and efficient type of detectors are the Solid State Crystalline. The photon passes through the patient and strikes the crystalline detector. The crystals change the energy to light, and the light is converted to an electrical signal. The other type of detector is the Xenon Gas Detectors. These are not commonly used today and they are inefficient. When the Xenon Gas Detector is hit with an x-ray, the gas is ionized. The ions migrate to a positive charge, charge plates, and create the electrical energy. All multi-row detectors in the past and all new detector systems have been built with the Crystalline Detectors.

34. C: The Data Acquisition System is a crucial process for Image Reconstruction. In short, the DAS measures the number of photons that strike the detectors, converts the information to a digital signal, and sends the signal to the computer. The measureable light or energy from the detectors is a very small signal that must pass through an Amplifier in the Gantry. Once the attenuation information has been amplified, it is sent to the computer system. The amplified signal is an analogue signal that must be digitized before it can be processed and stored on a computer. The ADC (analogue-to-digital converter) converts the analogue attenuation data into digital form. The now amplified digitized signal is sent as raw data to temporary storage to be reconstructed into an image by the Array Processor. The Array Processor reconstructs raw data into CT images. The data is sorted and goes through Filtered Back Projection and Convolution to produce a CT image viewed at the operator's console.

35. D: The development of Slip Rings allow for helical scanning capability. They are housed within the gantry. First and second generation CT scanners had cables that needed to be unwound to continue scanning. Continuous rotation scanners apply to third and fourth generation CT scanners when the development of slip rings eliminated the start and stop process with cables. The circular electrical conductive rings and brushes transmit energy across a rotating surface. Slip rings allow for faster scan times and continuous (helical) acquisition.

36. C: Single-Row Detector configurations have a single row of detectors arranged along the curves arc opposite the x-ray tube. First and Second Generation scanners contain single row detectors. MDCT are scanners with multiple parallel rows of detector elements arranged along a curved arc opposite the x-ray tube. This allows more than one slice to be acquired during each tube rotation. MDCT collects information from multiple anatomical slices in each rotation and allows for faster scan times, increased anatomical coverage, and thinner slices.

37. B: In order to establish the conditions that allow photon production, a high voltage needs to be applied across the two electrical terminals of the tube. The necessary high voltage is produced by the high voltage generator. It takes the low voltage and passes it through a series of wire coils to produce a very high voltage. High voltage is required to generate photons with enough energy to penetrate the patient's body with differentiated tissues in each slice.

38. A: When the cathode filament gets hotter, there is a tendency for electrons to escape from the filament and collide with the anode target. The temperature of the filament is indirectly controlled by tube current or mA. The technologist can adjust the mA at the CT operator's console. Tube current determines the number of x-ray photons produced by the CT x-ray tube. It also affects image quality and patient dose.

39. C: The path of the photons emitted from the x-ray tube need to be restricted so they don't spread out and irradiate more than the area of interest. Scatter radiation would also increase. Collimators restrict the path of x-rays. They are made out of radio-opaque materials which physically block x-rays. Two types of collimators are utilized in CT; they are pre-patient and post-patient collimators. Pre-Patient Collimators restrict the x-ray beam immediately after it exits the CT tube before the photons interact with the patient. It is a refinement of the x-ray beam thickness after it leaves the tube but before it enters the body. Pre-patient collimation also minimizes radiation dose to the patient by reducing scatter radiation.

40. A: The Data Acquisition System is a crucial process for Image Reconstruction. In short, the DAS measures the number of photons that strike the detectors, converts the information to a digital signal, and sends the signal to the computer. The measureable light or energy from the detectors is a very small signal that must pass through an Amplifier in the Gantry. Once the attenuation information has been amplified, it is sent to the computer system. The amplified signal is an analogue signal that must be digitized before it can be processed and stored on a computer. The ADC (analogue-to-digital converter) converts the analogue attenuation data into digital form. The now amplified digitized signal is sent as raw data to temporary storage to be reconstructed into an image by the Array Processor. The Array Processor reconstructs raw data into CT images. The data is sorted and goes through Filtered Back Projection and Convolution to produce a CT image viewed at the operator's console.

41. D: The power capacity of the generator determines the range of exposure techniques available on each particular CT system. CT generators produce kV in the 120-140kV range to increase the intensity and penetration of the x-ray beam. This will help to decrease patient dose. A higher kV will

also help reduce the heat to the x-ray tube by allowing the technologist to select a lower mA. This will help extend the life of the tube.

42. A: Tungsten is often used for the anode target material. It produces a higher intensity x-ray beam. Tungsten has an atomic number of 74.

43. C: CT tubes usually contain more than one size focal spot. The most common sizes are 0.5mm and 1.0mm. Smaller focal spots produce better spatial resolution (sharper images) because of reduced penumbra. They concentrate heat onto a smaller portion of the anode and therefore cannot tolerate as much heat. This makes tube cooling in CT a very important task.

44. B: Tube warm-ups are a part of the daily maintenance protocols. Most CT units will alert the technologist when the tube gets below a certain temperature and a tube warm-up will be recommended. Tube warm-ups prolong the life of the tube and allow for maximum mA capacity. They help produce high quality consistent images.

45. A: The Data Acquisition System is a crucial process for Image Reconstruction. In short, the DAS measures the number of photons that strike the detectors, converts the information to a digital signal, and sends the signal to the computer. The measureable light or energy from the detectors is a very small signal that must pass through an Amplifier in the Gantry. Once the attenuation information has been amplified, it is sent to the computer system. The amplified signal is an analogue signal that must be digitized before it can be processed and stored on a computer. The ADC (analogue-to-digital converter) converts the analogue attenuation data into digital form. The now amplified digitized signal is sent as raw data to temporary storage to be reconstructed into an image by the Array Processor. The Array Processor reconstructs raw data into CT images. The data is sorted and goes through Filtered Back Projection and Convolution to produce a CT image viewed at the operator's console.

46. B: 2nd Generation scanners contain a fan shaped x-ray beam, and a fixed anode. They have a translate-rotate scanning motion, and the detectors are in a straight line (linear detector array). 2nd Generation scanners took about 20 seconds to obtain one image. They do not have helical scanning ability or the benefit of a rotating anode.

47. C: 3rd Generation scanners are the most common technology used today. They have the ability for helical scans and a rotating anode. They have a fan beam geometry and translate-translate scanning motion. 3rd Generation technology has a multiple detector array along a curve and complete circular rotation of the detectors. They are fast, taking only 1 second per image.

48. C: EBCT has no x-ray tube. They have an electron gun that shoots out an electron beam to strike the anode. Neither the x-ray beam source nor the detectors move. It is considered ultrafast, and it was the preferred technology for cardiac CT until MDCT came along. Shortfalls in special resolution and high cost prevented this technology from being utilized for routine exams.

49. A: Conventional and helical scanning measure attenuation information through multiple projections. This information becomes raw data, and it requires further processing in the array processor to form the final CT image. Most CT systems today use Filtered Back Projection reconstruction to achieve the final image. There are two steps during this process. One is applying a filter to the raw data, and the other is Back Projection.

50. A: Back Projection is a process that occurs during Filtered Back Projection. It adds together the attenuation information collected from all the projections. That is still not enough information for a good image. The image will appear grainy with blurry edges. This is improved by applying a

reconstruction filter or kernel to the data. This process is called convolution. Its purpose is to enhance important characteristics of the image before back projection is performed. If back projection was applied to the raw data before convolution, the image would have blurry edges and a grainy appearance.

51. B: Smooth filters minimize the grainy image appearance. This is also known as noise. Sharp filters improve edge definition. With enough projections and the proper reconstruction filters applied, the back projection technique can accurately depict the original object in the final CT image.

52. D: Raw Data is all the information from the detector array prior to image reconstruction. Also called scan data, it refers to the computer data from the detectors that are waiting to be processed into a CT image. Raw Data has not assigned Hounsfield units or pixels. The process of using raw data to form an image is called image reconstruction. Once the raw data is processed so that each pixel is assigned a Hounsfield value, an image is created. This data is called image data.

53. B: Retrospective Reconstruction is the process of using raw data to later generate a new image. Raw data is required to generate new images in retrospective reconstruction. Image data cannot be used. Raw Data is lost once that portion of the raw data storage device is overwritten. Depending on how busy the particular scanner is, the raw data may only be available for a day or two or a few weeks. Retrospective Reconstruction is a valuable process enabling the technologist to change the algorithms, slice thickness, FOV, and other scan parameters.

54. C: Effective slice thickness is the thickness of the slice that is actually represented on the CT image. It is not the slice thickness selected by the collimator opening. In axial scanning, the selected slice thickness is equal to the effective slice thickness. In helical scanning, the effective slice thickness is usually wider than the selected slice thickness due to interpolation.

55. A: This imaging parameter is determined by the technologist. It determines where the helical slices will be reconstructed and if they will overlap. If the interval is equal to the thickness, the slices will be contiguous. If the interval is less than the thickness, the slices will overlap. There is no change to patient dose.

56. B: Post-processing allows the technologist to gain additional information from the patient's study without keeping the patient or using more radiation. Multiplanar reconstruction uses image data to change the orientation or plane of the original scan orientation. Images must be helically acquired for successful multiplanar reconstruction. The technologist can reconstruct the images to axial, coronal, sagittal, or oblique orientations.

57. D: Post-processing allows the technologist to gain additional information from the patient's study without keeping the patient or using more radiation. 3D reformatting utilizes thin slices and overlapping helically acquired image data to outline the outside of a structure. It includes only information from the surface of an object. There are many applications for 3D rendering depending on the equipment.

58. D: 3D reformatting utilizes thin slices and overlapping helically acquired image data to outline the outside of a structure. There are many applications for 3D rendering depending on the equipment. MIPs is a 3D technique that selects voxels with the highest value and displays them as the image reformat.

59. B: A pixel is a single picture element formed by the intersection of a row and column in the image grid to make the image matrix. The image matrix is the grid of rows and columns of pixels

that form the digital image. These grids and columns allow us to associate the location of a specific structure within the anatomical slice being imaged with a specific pixel.

60. A: A voxel is a volume element. It is a three dimensional cube of data acquired in CT. If the z-axis is taken into account, this results in a cube rather than a square (x and y-axis). The cube of data is referred to as a voxel.

61. C: Each CT slice represents a specific plane in the patient's body. The thickness of the plane is referred to as the z-axis. The technologist selects the slice thickness available on each specific scanner. When a slice thickness is selected, it limits the x-ray beam so it passes only through the specified volume. This will help lower scatter radiation and superimposition of other structures. Collimators are used to accomplish this limiting of the beam.

62. A: SFOV is the millimeters of anatomy over which the projection data is collected. It determines the area that data will be collected. It also determines the number of detectors collecting information. A cross section of a patient's anatomy should be completely contained within the SFOV. The CT numbers may be misrepresented on the final image if anatomy within the imaged slice is outside the SFOV.

63. B: The RFOV is the millimeters of information reconstructed and displayed in the final image. This is the FOV applied during reconstruction performed on the raw data. Increasing RFOV will make the anatomy appear smaller and make the image appear less noisy. The image may appear less noisy, but it is more difficult to see tiny structures. The RFOV has no effect on patient dose since it is done during the post scan process of reconstructing the data.

64. A: The matrix is a grid of rows and columns of pixels that form the digital image. These grids of rows and columns associate the location of a specific structure within the anatomical slice being imaged with a specific pixel. Increasing the matrix will yield smaller pixels, increase resolution, and increase the image noise. The matrix has no effect on patient dose.

65. D: Once the images have been reconstructed, the technologist or physician can adjust the brightness and contrast from the viewing computer. This is called windowing. After raw data is reconstructed, a CT number is assigned to represent the attenuation properties of the tissues in each pixel. The CT number corresponds to the Hounsfield Scale. The CT number for each pixel correlates to the gray scale. Water has a value of 0 and air has a value of -1000. Everything else falls within that scale based on attenuation. Windowing adjusts the brightness and contrast of these gray shades to optimize image quality. There are two window settings to adjust, window level and window width.

66. B: Windowing adjusts the brightness and contrast of these gray shades to optimize image quality. There are two window settings to adjust, window level and window width. Window width determines the range of CT numbers that occupy the full gray scale on the image monitor. Only the CT numbers within the specified range will be evenly distributed across the gray scale. The gray scale goes from black to bright white. Increasing the window width allows a larger range of CT numbers to be viewed within the gray scale. It will also make the image appear to have less contrast between tissues with similar CT numbers.

67. C: Godfrey N. Hounsfield is the English engineer who developed the first CT scanner. He received the Nobel Peace prize in 1979 with the physicist A.M Cormack. In 1972, the first clinical CT exam was performed.

68. A: A CT number is assigned to represent the attenuation properties of the tissues in each pixel. The CT number corresponds to the Hounsfield Scale. The CT number for each pixel correlates to the gray scale. Water has a value of 0 and air has a value of -1000. Everything else falls within that scale based on attenuation. The CT values of air and water are independent of the x-rays' energy, therefore they constitute fixed points for the CT scale. Lung tissue and fat are on the negative side of the scale because they have a lower attenuation coefficient due to less density. Most other body areas have positive CT values.

69. A: Picture Archiving and Communications Systems (PACS) allows electronic images and reports to be viewed and transmitted digitally. The universal format for PACS is DICOM. PACS eliminates traditional costly film retrieval and distribution. PACS can be utilized by all modalities and multiple clinical areas such as cardiology and laboratory. It provides hard copy replacement archiving and remote access. PACS also helps staff manage patient workflow.

70. B: Digital Imaging and Communications in Medicine (DICOM) enables digital communication between diagnostic and therapeutic systems within facilities and around the world. It is the universally adopted standard for medical image interchange. DICOM makes digital computer communications possible from multiple vendors. It improves cost-effectiveness. Medical images can be transferred quickly so treatment decisions can be made sooner.

71: B: The HIPAA act placed rules and regulations into law that protect the medical information of every patient in the United States. HIPAA is very specific about what privacy guidelines are to be used when medical images and files are moved through virtual channels. These are called HIPAA security requirements. Intense encryption of data and images passing over an internet connection are required.

72: D: Facilities must be able to recover medical images in the event of an error or disaster. HIPAA laws apply to all back-up methods with strict encryption and authorized access.

73. A: Online archiving is a medical image storage system that uses devices such as hard drives that make the information instantly accessible to the user. Off-line archiving is a storage system in which medical image data is stored in a less accessible location that requires manual extraction of data.

74. C: Noise is the grainy appearance seen on a final image. It becomes more apparent when there are insufficient photon numbers. We can adjust the number of photons which affects the noise level, but we cannot directly change noise. If the number of photons is increased, the patient dose is increased. There is a trade-off of dose increase for decreased noise.

75. B: Contrast is the ability to differentiate small differences in densities on the image. The energy level of the photon plays a key role in the contrast of the image. In CT the ability of the system to differentiate the contrasts of objects with similar densities is also called low-contrast resolution.

76. A: The technologist can make adjustments that will affect resolution. Pixel size, slice thickness, and reconstruction filter can be adjusted to help resolution. Also called spatial resolution, high-contrast resolution, and detail resolution.

77. D: Every CT scanner uses two set points on the CT value scale: air (1000 HU) and water (0 HU). These values are set and maintained by phantom testing. The goal of this regular testing is to ensure homogeneity or uniformity. Uniformity is maintaining a constant CT value for water over the entire cross section of an object.

78. B: CT image quality can typically be evaluated with a few criteria such as spatial resolution, low-contrast resolution, artifacts, and temporal resolution. Temporal resolution is the speed that the data can be acquired. The development of cardiac CT imaging has made temporal resolution a very important feature. The temporal resolution of a system is typically projected in milliseconds.

79. C: Temporal resolution is the speed that the data can be acquired. The speed is important because it helps to reduce or eliminate object motion artifacts. Temporal resolution is determined by the speed of gantry rotation, the number of detector channels, and the speed with which the system can record changing signals.

80. D: The digital image assigns a gray scale value to each pixel in the image based on the attenuation information of the beam from the tissues located in each slice. A CT number is assigned to represent the attenuation properties of the tissues in each pixel. The CT number correlates to the Hounsfield scale. The CT Number from the Hounsfield scale for each pixel correlates to a gray scale value.

81. B: Windowing the CT image to a diagnostically relevant range of CT values is accomplished by choosing the center and the width of the window. Lung tissue is best displayed with a center around -600 and width around 1700.

82. A: The relationship between CT numbers and the linear attenuation CT values of the scanned object is linearity. Linearity describes the performance of the CT system and the accuracy between the linear attenuation coefficient and the computer assigned CT number.

83. B: Quality Assurance protocols ensure that the CT system is producing the best possible imaging quality while utilizing the minimal amount of radiation dose to the patient. QA programs should entail tests that are performed on a regular basis, the results are recorded in a consistent format, and the documentation indicates that the parameters are within specified guidelines. Phantoms evaluate many aspects of image quality. Most phantoms are designed with a variety of components to evaluate a broad range of scanning parameters with one phantom. For example, the ACR CT accreditation phantom contains four modules.

84. A: Beam hardening occurs when lower energy photons are absorbed and leaving higher energy photons to strike the detectors. This causes dark bands or streaks across the image.

85. D: Beam hardening is a common artifact that occurs when there's an increase in the average energy of the x-ray beam as it penetrates tissue, causing dark bands or streaks through the CT image. To minimize, use correction algorithms, thin slices, and don't scan through very dense IV contrast.

86. B: PVA artifacts result from selecting slices that are much thicker than the anatomy and pathology that is being scanned. Different tissue attenuation values are averaged to produce one less accurate pixel reading. This appears as blurriness, incorrect CT numbers, and inconsistencies between image views. Using thinner slices can help reduce PVA artifacts.

87. C: Ring artifacts occur on third generation scanners. They appear on the CT image as ring or circle. It is considered a hardware artifact since it occurs from a faulty detector.

88. A: Tube arching occurs when a short circuit or surge of electrical current happens within the x-ray tube.

89. B: Artifacts produced by the edge gradient effect are mostly unavoidable, however thinner slices sometimes reduce the artifact. A common example of the edge gradient effect is when a barium sulfate lies next to air in the gastrointestinal tract. Sometimes a lower HU oral contrast like Volumen or water can eliminate the streaking in the GI tract.

90. A: Routine brain scans should begin at the skull base and scan through to the vertex. This will ensure that all brain structures will be included.

91. B: The posterior fossa houses the brain-stem and cerebellum. A MRI with gadolinium is the preferred imaging modality to best visualize the posterior fossa. CT can be utilized when an MRI is contraindicated.

92. C: Acoustic Neuromas are benign tumors. IACs for hearing loss to rule out an acoustic neuroma require the injection of IV contrast. IACs are done without IV contrast for cholesteatoma and mastoiditis. MRI with gadolinium is considered the imaging of choice for acoustic neuroma diagnosis.

93. B: The pituitary gland sends hormone signals to the endocrine glands. It is usually scanned C+. Axials and coronals are acquired from reconstructions or directly. Standard and sharp algorithms are utilized for detail. Axial views should include the sphenoid sinus through the dorsum sellum. Coronal views should begin at the anterior clinoid and through to the dorsum sella. Helical slice thickness varies from 0.5mm-2mm.

94. A: The optic nerves are best visualized in the axial image plane for CT of the orbits. It is also the best plane to evaluate the Lateral Rectus Muscles. Axial images should be obtained from the top of the Maxillary Sinuses through the Upper Orbital Rim. The patient should be head first and supine in the gantry with eyes closed to eliminate blinking motion.

95. C: Coronal images that are directly acquired for a sinus CT exam best visualize the air fluid levels. In order to directly acquire coronals, the patient must be scanned in the prone position. Some patients have difficulty assuming the prone position. Age, general health, and trauma sometimes limit a patient's ability to lie prone. In these situations, the patient will need to be scanned supine helically and coronal views reconstructed from the axial images.

96. A: The patient should not be placed prone, especially when there are obvious facial fractures. Supine head first is the appropriate patient position. Thin helical slices should be used since reconstructions will be necessary. Axial images will be directly acquired and coronal images will be reconstructed from that data. Some Radiologists also require sagittal plane or oblique reconstructions along with 3D.

97. D: Cellulitis is inflammation in the skin and deeper layers of the tissue. It is often caused by a bacterial infection. Symptoms include swelling, pain, redness, and heat to the infected areas. CT is one imaging modality used to diagnose the extent of the infection. IV contrast helps enhance the detail and extent of the infection.

98. A: Routine Brain CTs are often scanned serial/conventional rather than helical. This provides fine detail with no helical artifact issues. It gives the best image quality possible. Serial scanning also allows the technologist to angle the gantry so the scan can be done parallel to the base of the skull. The down side is a slower scan time. All CTAs must be scanned helically so reconstructions can be done and so the images can be acquired at a high speed.

99. B: Bolus timing is crucial for all CTAs. Bolus arrival times vary significantly between individuals. Cardiac output, IV gauge, speed of injection, area of interest, and general patient health all attribute to the timing of contrast arrival to the area of interest. A test bolus can be utilized with serial slices to determine the arrival time of contrast to the area of interest. Different manufacturers have bolus timing programs built into the software, such as Care Bolus and Smart Prep.

100. D: Recent practices favor angling parallel to the supraorbital meatal line rather than the orbital meatal line to avoid radiation to the radiosensitive lens of the eye. This is particularly important when imaging pediatrics.

101. A: Beam hardening is a common artifact that occurs when there's an increase in the average energy of the x-ray beam as it penetrates tissue causing dark bands or streaks through the CT image. To minimize, use correction algorithms, thin slices, and don't scan through very dense IV contrast. Increasing kVp and using thinner slices will help manage the beam hardening artifacts.

102. C: Tissue Plasminogen Activator (t-PA) is the only FDA approved treatment for acute ischemic stroke. A CT scan is vital prior to the administration of t-PA. A non-contrast CT scan must be performed to rule out a hemorrhagic bleed within the brain that may be causing similar symptoms as a stroke. To be effective, t-PA must be administered within 3 hours of the first stroke symptoms. CT must be available and speed is very important to getting a stroke diagnoses so t-PA can be administered safely.

103. B: This is the best window setting to view bone on a brain CT for trauma or postoperative patients.

104. D: Contrast media is not necessary when looking for a foreign body such as a chicken bone or glass. Contrast may obscure the foreign body. Salivary duct stones show up within the salivary duct as bright white. They are similar in density to IV contrast, so the injection of contrast media may obscure the stone. Normal thyroid tissue takes iodine from the blood stream and traps it within the cell to make thyroid hormone. Iodine contrast media will block iodine uptake by thyroid tissue for up to 6 months. This will reduce the benefit of future radioiodine therapy and iodine diagnostic scans. It is important not to delay tumor treatment for the thyroid for 6 months, so a non-contrast CT or MRI would be the best choice.

105. D: Having the patient refrain from swallowing during a neck CT will help to minimize motion. Breath holding may also help minimize motion.

106. A: When imaging the neck, it is important to allow sufficient time after contrast injection for the pathologic tissue, lymph nodes, and mucosa to enhance (or not enhance). However, the vasculature needs to remain opacified so neoplastic and inflammatory processes are detected. If the scan is too long after the contrast injection, the vessels will no longer be opacified, but the other tissues will be enhanced. One injection technique utilized is called a split bolus. This technique splits the total contrast dose. The first dose is given (usually half of volume), then a 2 minute delay, followed by a second bolus, and then the patient is scanned. This allows time for the structures that are slower to enhance to be opacified, and the second injection allows the vessels to be opacified as well.

107. C: IR is still considered the "gold standard" for the imaging of cervicocranial/cerebrovascular disease. IR can be time-consuming with an increased risk of permanent neurologic complications. The advances in multidetector CT systems and post-processing techniques have increased the use of CT for cerebrovascular evaluation. CT is non-invasive and widely available. It is also faster than IR.

108. B: The carotid arteries are the most common sites of TIAs (transient ischemic attack). They supply blood to the retinal artery. When there is a clot in the carotid, symptoms originate in the retina or cerebral hemisphere. Patients may experience visual symptoms. If the cerebral hemisphere is affected, problems with speech, paralysis, tingling, or numbness may be present. Carotid Ultrasound and CTA Brain and Neck are usually the imaging protocols followed to diagnose stroke.

109. D: Endoscopy is considered the standard for evaluation of laryngotracheobronchial conditions. Endoscopy allows for easy visualization and accurate diagnosis of mucosal and superficial lesions. The evaluation of deeper structures is capable only through CT imaging or MRI. CT imaging has become the most commonly used technique for general laryngeal imaging. CT provides fast and accurate results in any trauma scenario. It is also readily accessible in most areas. This will help the provider diagnose and treat the patient quickly and accurately.

110. C: Lung cancer often metastasizes to the adrenal glands. It is important for cancer staging to scan from the sternal notch through to the adrenal glands. This will ensure all important lung anatomy is covered.

111. C: A fast CT image acquisition allows the entire lungs to be scanned during a single breath hold. Airway imaging is routinely performed with inspiration and expiration techniques. This provides the Radiologist with two series to evaluate the airways and diagnose the extent of pathology.

112. A: HRCT is a CT Chest protocol used to evaluate the lung parenchyma. In addition to the thin slices, selected spatial resolution is optimized by selecting an edge-enhancing algorithm. Most HRCT protocols include a series of scans. For example, some facilities may scan a routine chest CT with 5mm slices and a stacked 10mm series with edge algorithm. Some facilities will scan at full inspiration and for certain diseases an expiration series will also be scanned.

113. B: The Systemic Vascular Route of Injection is as follows: Accessed Vein, Brachial, Axillary, Subclavian, SVC, Right Atrium, Right Ventricle, Pulmonary Arteries, Left Atrium, Left Ventricle, Aorta, and back to Venous and Heart. The Vascular Route of Injection is crucial for bolus timing, especially within the chest. Cardiac CT imaging is entirely dependent on the bolus timing. Knowing the route of contrast is important for a technologist to accurately time the scan to acquire images at the peak enhancement for a specific area of interest.

114. B: CT Venography (CTV) may be done to assess for venous thrombosis in the pelvis and lower extremities. These are common sites for clots to form and travel to upper vasculature causing heart attack and stroke. A second scan series is performed after the CTA with a delayed venous phase (about 180 seconds after the injection of IV contrast). A scan is done from the iliac crests through both knees.

115. B: The advances made with MDCT have improved spatial and temporal resolution, especially with all CTA procedures. Even with these advances, strategies to eliminate heart muscle motion artifact during CTA Cardiac procedures became important. Obviously, we can't stop the heart from beating for a CT exam. One development was the administration of Beta-Blockers to temporarily lower a patient's heart rate and help make it regular. Ideally, the heart rate should be less than 65 bpm. A lower heart rate allows the technologist more time in between beats to complete the crucial part of the cardiac CTA. The second technique is called cardiac gating. ECG leads are placed on the patient, and the ECG machine is connected to the CT gantry. The gating attempts to identify the lowest cardiac motion and acquire images only in those portions of the cardiac cycle. It guides the technologist in planning out the best possible time to start the bolus and acquire the images. If a

cardiac CTA is not performed with perfect bolus, timing, and heart rate, the exam is of little use for an accurate diagnosis. The Technologist's skill is very important during these procedures along with patient cooperation.

116. A: A patient's respirations affect the lung bases more than the lung apices. Breathing motion tends to affect the peripheral and smaller arteries more than the larger centrally located arteries. A caudal-cranial scan direction is especially helpful when a patient is unable to hold their breath for the entire scan. If they do have to breathe during image acquisition, the motion will be less noticeable in the lung apices towards the end of the scan. Since PEs often cause shortness of breath, it can be expected that the patient will have difficultly holding their breath for the entire scan.

117. D: The experience and knowledge of the CT technologist is so important in producing the best possible CTA. The dose, rate, and timing of the IV contrast are critical in producing a diagnostic CTA examination. The chest is a difficult area to image due to breathing and cardiac motion. The various densities within the mediastinum also produce some imaging complications. As with all CTAs, the contrast timing, rate, and dose are all important factors to adjust for the best possible CTA exam. Contrast Bolus Tracking and Triggering all assist the technologist with the contrast timing and peak vascular enhancement commencing with image acquisition.

118. A: Beam-hardening is a common artifact that occurs when there's an increase in the average energy of the x-ray beam as it penetrates tissue, causing dark bands or streaks through the CT image. To minimize, use correction algorithms, thin slices, and don't scan through very dense IV contrast. A saline injection after the contrast injection will reduce or eliminate beam-hardening artifacts from the dense contrast in the superior vena cava. This density in the SVC might obscure small emboli in certain vessels like the right upper lobe and right main pulmonary arteries.

119. A: Thoracic imaging can be challenging due to a continuously beating heart and multiple vascular structures. The advances made with MDCT have improved spatial and temporal resolution especially with thoracic procedures. Spatial resolution is the CT systems ability to resolve with detail small objects that are very close together. Temporal resolution is how quickly data is acquired. It is controlled by the speed of gantry rotation, the number of detectors in the system, and how quickly the system can record changing signals.

120. C: This test is ordered to help rule out thrombus. D-Dimer results may be used to determine if further testing is necessary to help diagnose hypercoagulability. It is considered an inexpensive blood test that is used as a screening to determine if a CT, Ultrasound, or Nuclear Medicine VQ-Scan needs to be performed. If D-Dimer values are within the normal range, there is a low likelihood of PE. However, an abnormal D-Dimer does not confirm the presence of thrombus in the body. There are multiple contributing factors that can raise the D-Dimer value. An elevated value indicates the need for further testing.

121. D: The main pulmonary artery divides into left and right pulmonary arteries. They can be closely followed by observing the subdivision of the bronchial tree. This helps the viewer easily identify the pulmonary artery on cross-sectional images.

122. B: The density effects from gravity are more pronounced on expiratory HRCT of the chest. Some HRCT protocols include an inspiratory prone series to help differentiate actual disease from densities that are affected by gravity mimicking disease. These protocols are usually determined by the Radiologist.

123. B: Axial.

124. C: Coronal.

125. B: Main Pulmonary Artery.

126. A: Sagittal.

127. A: There are 3 phases of contrast enhancement: Bolus, Non-Equilibrium, and Equilibrium Phases. The first phase of enhancement is the Bolus phase. This is an optimal phase for CTAs. There is a significant density difference between the abdominal aorta and IVC. The second phase is the Non-Equilibrium phase. During this phase, the bolus disperses into the capillaries and then into the veins. The two phases of enhancement within this phase are the Hepatic Arterial (typically about 25 seconds post-contrast injection) and Portal Venous. The Non-Equilibrium phase provides the best differentiation of structures in soft tissue, like the liver and pancreas. The third phase is Equilibrium. During this phase, the concentration of contrast in the veins and arteries are similar and soft tissue differentiation becomes diminished.

128. C: Overall patient health and general compliance will affect how much volume will be consumed. Some patients are vomiting and too nauseous to drink the required volume of oral prep. Other patients simply refuse to drink the oral prep. The greater the volume of oral contrast consumption will provide the best bowel opacification. At least 600 mL of oral contrast is desired for the best bowel opacification.

129. B: Most Abdomen CT scans require oral contrast (either barium sulfate or a water-soluble agent). Oral contrast helps visualize the intestinal lumen and it distends the intestinal tract. However, its use is so important because it helps the Radiologist differentiate normal fluid filled loops of bowel from an abnormal mass or abscess.

130. C: This is the best window setting to view soft tissue abdominal anatomy for most patients.

131. B: A hemangioma is a benign tumor that is often discovered incidentally during other imaging exams like ultrasound. Unenhanced hemangiomas appear as a well-defined hypo dense mass. After the lesion is enhanced, it begins a progressive pooling of contrast beginning at the periphery. Often delayed images are done to confirm the lesions being uniformly enhanced after 10-15 minutes past injection.

132. A: CT is the imaging modality of choice for the best visualization of the pancreas. It provides more reliable overall diagnostic information than other imaging modalities. IV contrast helps provide a more detailed image of the pancreas. Water or other low-attenuation oral preps help to distinguish the duodenum form the pancreas without obscuring small stones.

133. C: CTU protocols are fairly new. They were designed to provide the most thorough CT evaluations of the upper and lower urinary system, or the kidneys, ureters, and bladder. There are many different protocols used based on the ordering of Urologists or the reading of Radiologists. A typical CTU protocol may be a non-contrast abdomen and pelvis, arterial renal abdomen, portal venous abdomen and pelvis, and excretory delayed abdomen and pelvis. Sometimes the protocol is based on pathology or symptoms. A single bolus injection or a split bolus injection may also be utilized. The split bolus injection combines two phases and therefore reduces radiation to the patient. This method is becoming more popular due to dose reduction.

134. D: Exact timing of IV contrast is patient dependent, so bolus tracking software is commonly used to time exams. The average scan delay for most patients when imaging the portal venous

phase of the liver is a scan delay time of 65-75 seconds. For a biphasic liver, the arterial scan delay time is usually 20-25 seconds.

135. B: Non-contrast helical abdomen and pelvic CT has become the standard technique for the evaluation suspected urinary tract calculi. IV and/or oral contrast could obscure the stone since the density of the contrast agents is similar to the densities of the calcification.

136. D: Bi-Phasic liver scanning is usually done for any hyper vascular lesions or vascular hepatic anatomy. The liver receives about 25% of its blood supply from the hepatic artery and the remaining percentage of blood from the portal vein. There are several possible phases of contrast enhancement for the liver due to its dual blood supply. Different types of masses will enhance differently depending on that tumor's particular blood supply.

137. B: The adrenals are part of the endocrine system. They are retroperitoneal like the kidneys. Adrenal masses are common, and CT is the imaging modality of choice to best visualize them. Adrenal masses are often an incidental finding. CT is astute in diagnosing benign adrenal masses from malignant or metastasis masses. This is accomplished by measuring the attenuation values. This is done by evaluating the degree to which the IV contrast is washed out on the delayed imaging. A non-contrast adrenal CT is necessary to determine the unenhanced HU of the adrenal glands.

138. A: 75-85 seconds.

139. D: All CTAs are well-timed vascular helical exams. The IV contrast enhances the vessels and allows visualization of abnormalities. No oral prep is required for a CTA for the Aorta, but IV contrast is a must. A proper delay time must be used to guarantee that, from the first to the last rotation of helical acquisition, there will be contrast in the vessels of interest. In order to get the best possible images on all CTAs, the following list is best. The patient should have an excellent IV site with a minimum of a 20G needle. A fast injection rate is necessary, 5cc/second is a good choice if possible with IV access. A dense contrast media should be used with no dilution, preferably over 300 concentrations. In addition to the above criteria, the scan should occur during peak vessel enhancement by utilizing a test injection or bolus timing software.

140. C: Depending on the scanner and the patient's habitus, the 200-300 mAs range is commonly utilized to image a routine abdomen CT. If the technologist selected thinner slices, the technique may need to be increased to reduce noise.

141. C: Rectal contrast is utilized to visualize the distal colon in male and female Pelvic CT exams. It also helps to differentiate the colon from other pelvic anatomy. Rectal contrast is often used when a rectal pathology is suspected or a patient cannot tolerate the oral prep.

142. D: Body Imaging is routinely scanned helical. Helical images cannot be acquired with a tilt on the gantry. A straight axial plane is utilized for body imaging.

143. A: This will ensure that the entire pelvic cavity and bone structures of the pelvis will be imaged.

144. A: The left and right Common Iliac Arteries begin when the abdominal aorta bifurcates at the level of L-4.

145. D: Aorta.

146. A: Kidney.

147. B: Bladder.

148. C: McBurney's is located in the right lower quadrant of the abdomen/pelvic region. Classic appendicitis presents as right lower quadrant pain. Tenderness is often most intense near McBurney's point. The attending physician will push down on this area and lift up. If pain or tenderness is present on the rebound, this is known as McBurney's sign. It is a common indicator of appendicitis.

149. A: Acute Appendicitis can often be diagnosed when the CT images display a dilated and non-contrast opacified appendix. There may also be soft tissue stranding or inflammation around the adjacent tissues. Sometimes an appendicolith may also be present.

150. B: Patient size and scanner type may influence the amount of IV contrast administered. A patient's renal function may also dictate lowering the amount of contrast media injected. On average, a typical amount of contrast necessary for proper vessel and organ opacification is between 65 and 100 cc.

151. D: A patient should be Supine for an Abdomen and Pelvic CT. They should be placed feet first into the gantry with their arms above their head.

152. A: Adenomas tend to have a homogenous density with smooth margins. Any homogenous adrenal mass presented on an unenhanced CT image with a Hounsfield measurement less than 10HU is considered benign. However, lesions which measure more than 10HU cannot be assumed to be malignant. Further CT testing with contrast is usually required. If those results are still inconclusive, a biopsy will need to be performed.

153. B: The Portal Vein provides blood supply to the liver.

154. C: Musculoskeletal protocols and techniques are tailored to the individual patient and region of interest. Patients should be positioned so both sides are as symmetric as possible. A lateral and AP scout are recommended. It is important to scan long bones with the CT plane perpendicular to the long axis for the best images possible. This is not always possible when a patient has a fracture is in a hard cast.

155. B: CT images of the foot/ankle can be displayed in many different imaging planes. Some planes can be acquired directly (without reformatting) by positioning the patient in a particular way. The axial plane is parallel to the plantar surface of the foot. This can be acquired directly by positioning the patient feet first in the gantry with the toes pointing straight up with no gantry tilt.

156. A: To obtain a direct oblique coronal plane on foot/ankle CT exams, the patient should be positioned with knees bent and feet flat on the scan table. The gantry is angled 20-30 degrees perpendicular to the subtalar joint. This will acquire the scan data in a direct oblique coronal plane.

157. C: A CT arthrogram of the shoulder utilizes an injection of contrast media and air directly into the joint space. The patient is then scanned in CT. CT arthrography will help evaluate the joint space and other joint structures. It will also help diagnose loose bodies within the joint space.

158. B: Intrathecal contrast is administered within the spine to evaluate disk disease. The contrast is usually injected by a Radiologist under fluoroscopy. A delay of 1-3 hours is recommended to allow the contrast time dilute with spinal fluid. The spinal scan shouldn't be performed when the

contrast is too dense. Sometimes the technologist has the patient roll a few times to coat the spinal column before scanning the patient.

159. D: CT scans of the extremities allow the ability to show precise information about the presence, location, orientation, and relationship of a fracture. It also depicts boney tumors. When soft tissue structures like cartilage, ligaments, and muscles need to be visualized, an MRI is necessary.

160. B: Thinner acquired CT slices will equal better reconstructions. Musculoskeletal imaging requires data to be viewed in different planes. Coronal, sagittal, and axial planes are often desired. Helical thin slices in the 0.625mm-1.25mm ranges will allow for the best reconstructions and 3D images.

161. A: Calcaneus.

162. B: L-3.

163. A: Femoral Head.

164. C: Patella.

165. A: Scapula.

How to Overcome Test Anxiety

Just the thought of taking a test is enough to make most people a little nervous. A test is an important event that can have a long-term impact on your future, so it's important to take it seriously and it's natural to feel anxious about performing well. But just because anxiety is normal, that doesn't mean that it's helpful in test taking, or that you should simply accept it as part of your life. Anxiety can have a variety of effects. These effects can be mild, like making you feel slightly nervous, or severe, like blocking your ability to focus or remember even a simple detail.

If you experience test anxiety—whether severe or mild—it's important to know how to beat it. To discover this, first you need to understand what causes test anxiety.

Causes of Test Anxiety

While we often think of anxiety as an uncontrollable emotional state, it can actually be caused by simple, practical things. One of the most common causes of test anxiety is that a person does not feel adequately prepared for their test. This feeling can be the result of many different issues such as poor study habits or lack of organization, but the most common culprit is time management. Starting to study too late, failing to organize your study time to cover all of the material, or being distracted while you study will mean that you're not well prepared for the test. This may lead to cramming the night before, which will cause you to be physically and mentally exhausted for the test. Poor time management also contributes to feelings of stress, fear, and hopelessness as you realize you are not well prepared but don't know what to do about it.

Other times, test anxiety is not related to your preparation for the test but comes from unresolved fear. This may be a past failure on a test, or poor performance on tests in general. It may come from comparing yourself to others who seem to be performing better or from the stress of living up to expectations. Anxiety may be driven by fears of the future—how failure on this test would affect your educational and career goals. These fears are often completely irrational, but they can still negatively impact your test performance.

Review Video: 3 Reasons You Have Test Anxiety
Visit mometrix.com/academy and enter code: 428468

Elements of Test Anxiety

As mentioned earlier, test anxiety is considered to be an emotional state, but it has physical and mental components as well. Sometimes you may not even realize that you are suffering from test anxiety until you notice the physical symptoms. These can include trembling hands, rapid heartbeat, sweating, nausea, and tense muscles. Extreme anxiety may lead to fainting or vomiting. Obviously, any of these symptoms can have a negative impact on testing. It is important to recognize them as soon as they begin to occur so that you can address the problem before it damages your performance.

> **Review Video: 3 Ways to Tell You Have Test Anxiety**
> Visit mometrix.com/academy and enter code: 927847

The mental components of test anxiety include trouble focusing and inability to remember learned information. During a test, your mind is on high alert, which can help you recall information and stay focused for an extended period of time. However, anxiety interferes with your mind's natural processes, causing you to blank out, even on the questions you know well. The strain of testing during anxiety makes it difficult to stay focused, especially on a test that may take several hours. Extreme anxiety can take a huge mental toll, making it difficult not only to recall test information but even to understand the test questions or pull your thoughts together.

> **Review Video: How Test Anxiety Affects Memory**
> Visit mometrix.com/academy and enter code: 609003

Effects of Test Anxiety

Test anxiety is like a disease—if left untreated, it will get progressively worse. Anxiety leads to poor performance, and this reinforces the feelings of fear and failure, which in turn lead to poor performances on subsequent tests. It can grow from a mild nervousness to a crippling condition. If allowed to progress, test anxiety can have a big impact on your schooling, and consequently on your future.

Test anxiety can spread to other parts of your life. Anxiety on tests can become anxiety in any stressful situation, and blanking on a test can turn into panicking in a job situation. But fortunately, you don't have to let anxiety rule your testing and determine your grades. There are a number of relatively simple steps you can take to move past anxiety and function normally on a test and in the rest of life.

> **Review Video: How Test Anxiety Impacts Your Grades**
> Visit mometrix.com/academy and enter code: 939819

Physical Steps for Beating Test Anxiety

While test anxiety is a serious problem, the good news is that it can be overcome. It doesn't have to control your ability to think and remember information. While it may take time, you can begin taking steps today to beat anxiety.

Just as your first hint that you may be struggling with anxiety comes from the physical symptoms, the first step to treating it is also physical. Rest is crucial for having a clear, strong mind. If you are tired, it is much easier to give in to anxiety. But if you establish good sleep habits, your body and mind will be ready to perform optimally, without the strain of exhaustion. Additionally, sleeping well helps you to retain information better, so you're more likely to recall the answers when you see the test questions.

Getting good sleep means more than going to bed on time. It's important to allow your brain time to relax. Take study breaks from time to time so it doesn't get overworked, and don't study right before bed. Take time to rest your mind before trying to rest your body, or you may find it difficult to fall asleep.

> **Review Video: The Importance of Sleep for Your Brain**
> Visit mometrix.com/academy and enter code: 319338

Along with sleep, other aspects of physical health are important in preparing for a test. Good nutrition is vital for good brain function. Sugary foods and drinks may give a burst of energy but this burst is followed by a crash, both physically and emotionally. Instead, fuel your body with protein and vitamin-rich foods.

Also, drink plenty of water. Dehydration can lead to headaches and exhaustion, especially if your brain is already under stress from the rigors of the test. Particularly if your test is a long one, drink water during the breaks. And if possible, take an energy-boosting snack to eat between sections.

> **Review Video: How Diet Can Affect your Mood**
> Visit mometrix.com/academy and enter code: 624317

Along with sleep and diet, a third important part of physical health is exercise. Maintaining a steady workout schedule is helpful, but even taking 5-minute study breaks to walk can help get your blood pumping faster and clear your head. Exercise also releases endorphins, which contribute to a positive feeling and can help combat test anxiety.

When you nurture your physical health, you are also contributing to your mental health. If your body is healthy, your mind is much more likely to be healthy as well. So take time to rest, nourish your body with healthy food and water, and get moving as much as possible. Taking these physical steps will make you stronger and more able to take the mental steps necessary to overcome test anxiety.

> **Review Video: How to Stay Healthy and Prevent Test Anxiety**
> Visit mometrix.com/academy and enter code: 877894

Mental Steps for Beating Test Anxiety

Working on the mental side of test anxiety can be more challenging, but as with the physical side, there are clear steps you can take to overcome it. As mentioned earlier, test anxiety often stems from lack of preparation, so the obvious solution is to prepare for the test. Effective studying may be the most important weapon you have for beating test anxiety, but you can and should employ several other mental tools to combat fear.

First, boost your confidence by reminding yourself of past success—tests or projects that you aced. If you're putting as much effort into preparing for this test as you did for those, there's no reason you should expect to fail here. Work hard to prepare; then trust your preparation.

Second, surround yourself with encouraging people. It can be helpful to find a study group, but be sure that the people you're around will encourage a positive attitude. If you spend time with others who are anxious or cynical, this will only contribute to your own anxiety. Look for others who are motivated to study hard from a desire to succeed, not from a fear of failure.

Third, reward yourself. A test is physically and mentally tiring, even without anxiety, and it can be helpful to have something to look forward to. Plan an activity following the test, regardless of the outcome, such as going to a movie or getting ice cream.

When you are taking the test, if you find yourself beginning to feel anxious, remind yourself that you know the material. Visualize successfully completing the test. Then take a few deep, relaxing breaths and return to it. Work through the questions carefully but with confidence, knowing that you are capable of succeeding.

Developing a healthy mental approach to test taking will also aid in other areas of life. Test anxiety affects more than just the actual test—it can be damaging to your mental health and even contribute to depression. It's important to beat test anxiety before it becomes a problem for more than testing.

> **Review Video:** Test Anxiety and Depression
> Visit mometrix.com/academy and enter code: 904704

Study Strategy

Being prepared for the test is necessary to combat anxiety, but what does being prepared look like? You may study for hours on end and still not feel prepared. What you need is a strategy for test prep. The next few pages outline our recommended steps to help you plan out and conquer the challenge of preparation.

Step 1: Scope Out the Test

Learn everything you can about the format (multiple choice, essay, etc.) and what will be on the test. Gather any study materials, course outlines, or sample exams that may be available. Not only will this help you to prepare, but knowing what to expect can help to alleviate test anxiety.

Step 2: Map Out the Material

Look through the textbook or study guide and make note of how many chapters or sections it has. Then divide these over the time you have. For example, if a book has 15 chapters and you have five days to study, you need to cover three chapters each day. Even better, if you have the time, leave an extra day at the end for overall review after you have gone through the material in depth.

If time is limited, you may need to prioritize the material. Look through it and make note of which sections you think you already have a good grasp on, and which need review. While you are studying, skim quickly through the familiar sections and take more time on the challenging parts. Write out your plan so you don't get lost as you go. Having a written plan also helps you feel more in control of the study, so anxiety is less likely to arise from feeling overwhelmed at the amount to cover. A sample plan may look like this:

- Day 1: Skim chapters 1–4, study chapter 5 (especially pages 31–33)
- Day 2: Study chapters 6–7, skim chapters 8–9
- Day 3: Skim chapter 10, study chapters 11–12 (especially pages 87–90)
- Day 4: Study chapters 13–15
- Day 5: Overall review (focus most on chapters 5, 6, and 12), take practice test

Step 3: Gather Your Tools

Decide what study method works best for you. Do you prefer to highlight in the book as you study and then go back over the highlighted portions? Or do you type out notes of the important information? Or is it helpful to make flashcards that you can carry with you? Assemble the pens, index cards, highlighters, post-it notes, and any other materials you may need so you won't be distracted by getting up to find things while you study.

If you're having a hard time retaining the information or organizing your notes, experiment with different methods. For example, try color-coding by subject with colored pens, highlighters, or post-it notes. If you learn better by hearing, try recording yourself reading your notes so you can listen while in the car, working out, or simply sitting at your desk. Ask a friend to quiz you from your flashcards, or try teaching someone the material to solidify it in your mind.

Step 4: Create Your Environment

It's important to avoid distractions while you study. This includes both the obvious distractions like visitors and the subtle distractions like an uncomfortable chair (or a too-comfortable couch that makes you want to fall asleep). Set up the best study environment possible: good lighting and a comfortable work area. If background music helps you focus, you may want to turn it on, but otherwise keep the room quiet. If you are using a computer to take notes, be sure you don't have any other windows open, especially applications like social media, games, or anything else that could distract you. Silence your phone and turn off notifications. Be sure to keep water close by so you stay hydrated while you study (but avoid unhealthy drinks and snacks).

Also, take into account the best time of day to study. Are you freshest first thing in the morning? Try to set aside some time then to work through the material. Is your mind clearer in the afternoon or evening? Schedule your study session then. Another method is to study at the same time of day that you will take the test, so that your brain gets used to working on the material at that time and will be ready to focus at test time.

Step 5: Study!

Once you have done all the study preparation, it's time to settle into the actual studying. Sit down, take a few moments to settle your mind so you can focus, and begin to follow your study plan. Don't give in to distractions or let yourself procrastinate. This is your time to prepare so you'll be ready to fearlessly approach the test. Make the most of the time and stay focused.

Of course, you don't want to burn out. If you study too long you may find that you're not retaining the information very well. Take regular study breaks. For example, taking five minutes out of every hour to walk briskly, breathing deeply and swinging your arms, can help your mind stay fresh.

As you get to the end of each chapter or section, it's a good idea to do a quick review. Remind yourself of what you learned and work on any difficult parts. When you feel that you've mastered the material, move on to the next part. At the end of your study session, briefly skim through your notes again.

But while review is helpful, cramming last minute is NOT. If at all possible, work ahead so that you won't need to fit all your study into the last day. Cramming overloads your brain with more information than it can process and retain, and your tired mind may struggle to recall even previously learned information when it is overwhelmed with last-minute study. Also, the urgent nature of cramming and the stress placed on your brain contribute to anxiety. You'll be more likely to go to the test feeling unprepared and having trouble thinking clearly.

So don't cram, and don't stay up late before the test, even just to review your notes at a leisurely pace. Your brain needs rest more than it needs to go over the information again. In fact, plan to finish your studies by noon or early afternoon the day before the test. Give your brain the rest of the day to relax or focus on other things, and get a good night's sleep. Then you will be fresh for the test and better able to recall what you've studied.

Step 6: Take a practice test

Many courses offer sample tests, either online or in the study materials. This is an excellent resource to check whether you have mastered the material, as well as to prepare for the test format and environment.

Check the test format ahead of time: the number of questions, the type (multiple choice, free response, etc.), and the time limit. Then create a plan for working through them. For example, if you have 30 minutes to take a 60-question test, your limit is 30 seconds per question. Spend less time on the questions you know well so that you can take more time on the difficult ones.

If you have time to take several practice tests, take the first one open book, with no time limit. Work through the questions at your own pace and make sure you fully understand them. Gradually work up to taking a test under test conditions: sit at a desk with all study materials put away and set a timer. Pace yourself to make sure you finish the test with time to spare and go back to check your answers if you have time.

After each test, check your answers. On the questions you missed, be sure you understand why you missed them. Did you misread the question (tests can use tricky wording)? Did you forget the information? Or was it something you hadn't learned? Go back and study any shaky areas that the practice tests reveal.

Taking these tests not only helps with your grade, but also aids in combating test anxiety. If you're already used to the test conditions, you're less likely to worry about it, and working through tests until you're scoring well gives you a confidence boost. Go through the practice tests until you feel comfortable, and then you can go into the test knowing that you're ready for it.

Test Tips

On test day, you should be confident, knowing that you've prepared well and are ready to answer the questions. But aside from preparation, there are several test day strategies you can employ to maximize your performance.

First, as stated before, get a good night's sleep the night before the test (and for several nights before that, if possible). Go into the test with a fresh, alert mind rather than staying up late to study.

Try not to change too much about your normal routine on the day of the test. It's important to eat a nutritious breakfast, but if you normally don't eat breakfast at all, consider eating just a protein bar. If you're a coffee drinker, go ahead and have your normal coffee. Just make sure you time it so that the caffeine doesn't wear off right in the middle of your test. Avoid sugary beverages, and drink enough water to stay hydrated but not so much that you need a restroom break 10 minutes into the test. If your test isn't first thing in the morning, consider going for a walk or doing a light workout before the test to get your blood flowing.

Allow yourself enough time to get ready, and leave for the test with plenty of time to spare so you won't have the anxiety of scrambling to arrive in time. Another reason to be early is to select a good seat. It's helpful to sit away from doors and windows, which can be distracting. Find a good seat, get out your supplies, and settle your mind before the test begins.

When the test begins, start by going over the instructions carefully, even if you already know what to expect. Make sure you avoid any careless mistakes by following the directions.

Then begin working through the questions, pacing yourself as you've practiced. If you're not sure on an answer, don't spend too much time on it, and don't let it shake your confidence. Either skip it and come back later, or eliminate as many wrong answers as possible and guess among the remaining ones. Don't dwell on these questions as you continue—put them out of your mind and focus on what lies ahead.

Be sure to read all of the answer choices, even if you're sure the first one is the right answer. Sometimes you'll find a better one if you keep reading. But don't second-guess yourself if you do immediately know the answer. Your gut instinct is usually right. Don't let test anxiety rob you of the information you know.

If you have time at the end of the test (and if the test format allows), go back and review your answers. Be cautious about changing any, since your first instinct tends to be correct, but make sure you didn't misread any of the questions or accidentally mark the wrong answer choice. Look over any you skipped and make an educated guess.

At the end, leave the test feeling confident. You've done your best, so don't waste time worrying about your performance or wishing you could change anything. Instead, celebrate the successful completion of this test. And finally, use this test to learn how to deal with anxiety even better next time.

> **Review Video:** 5 Tips to Beat Test Anxiety
> Visit mometrix.com/academy and enter code: 570656

Important Qualification

Not all anxiety is created equal. If your test anxiety is causing major issues in your life beyond the classroom or testing center, or if you are experiencing troubling physical symptoms related to your anxiety, it may be a sign of a serious physiological or psychological condition. If this sounds like your situation, we strongly encourage you to seek professional help.

Thank You

We at Mometrix would like to extend our heartfelt thanks to you, our friend and patron, for allowing us to play a part in your journey. It is a privilege to serve people from all walks of life who are unified in their commitment to building the best future they can for themselves.

The preparation you devote to these important testing milestones may be the most valuable educational opportunity you have for making a real difference in your life. We encourage you to put your heart into it—that feeling of succeeding, overcoming, and yes, conquering will be well worth the hours you've invested.

We want to hear your story, your struggles and your successes, and if you see any opportunities for us to improve our materials so we can help others even more effectively in the future, please share that with us as well. **The team at Mometrix would be absolutely thrilled to hear from you!** So please, send us an email (support@mometrix.com) and let's stay in touch.

If you'd like some additional help, check out these other resources we offer for your exam:

http://MometrixFlashcards.com/CT

Additional Bonus Material

Due to our efforts to try to keep this book to a manageable length, we've created a link that will give you access to all of your additional bonus material.

Please visit **https://www.mometrix.com/bonus948/ct** to access the information.